Praise for *Sex for Grownups*

"As a woman hovering on the precipice of 50 and a cosmetic dermatologist to many aging women, I personally and professionally welcome Dr. Lynn's contribution. Along with her individualized and insightful therapeutic approaches, Dr. Lynn's assessment that every female is 'an agent of change' serves as a useful tag line to guide us through the journey."

**—Tina Alster, M.D., director of
the Washington Institute of Dermatologic Laser Surgery**

"If you are young at heart, and you want to feel the fire Dr. Lynn's book is for you! It will take you from the Alpha to the Omega and you will enjoy the journey! It belongs on every boomer's nightstand."

—JC Hayward, vice president, WUSA-TV9

"Life after 50 can be a wonderful and surprising cascade of self-discovery. That goes for your sex life, especially, and by examining what's going on in your head as well as your body parts. Dr. Dorree Lynn's new book reveals the path to satisfying lifelong intimacy."

**—Daniel J. Kadlec, coauthor of
With Purpose and *The Power Years***

"Sex, intimacy, and aging have long been ignored by health professionals and the public. Dr. Dorree Lynn's inviting book for men, women, and couples over 50 brings empowerment for enjoying the pleasures of eroticism and love-making throughout life."

**—Barry McCarthy, Ph.D., professor of psychology at
American University and coauthor of
Men's Sexual Health and 10 other books on sex**

"Dr. Dorree offers wise counsel and practical advice for how to turn the inevitable alterations of aging to our erotic advantage. Finally, a book that tells it like is—sex can get better as we get older! And Dr. Dorree tells us how!"

—**Sheri Winston, CNM, RN, BSN, LMT,**
wholistic sexuality teacher, founder of the Center for the
Intimate Arts, and author of *Women's Anatomy of Arousal*

"Hang on everyone! Help is on the way. Dr. Dorree Lynn promises to rescue all of us and not a moment too soon."

—**Kitty Kelley, bestselling author of**
The Family: The Real Story of The Bush Dynasty

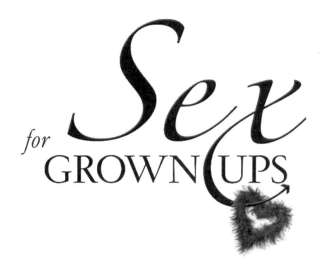

Sex
for GROWN UPS

Dr. Dorree Reveals the
Truth, Lies, and Must-Tries for
Great Sex After 50

Dorree Lynn, Ph.D., with Cindy Spitzer

Health Communications, Inc.
Deerfield Beach, Florida

www.hcibooks.com

Library of Congress Cataloging-in-Publication Data

Lynn, Dorree.
  Sex for grownups : Dr. Dorree reveals the truth, lies, and must-tries for great sex after 50 / Dorree Lynn, with Cindy Spitzer.
    p. cm.
  Includes bibliographical references and index.
  ISBN-13: 978-0-7573-1464-3
  ISBN-10: 0-7573-1464-3
  1. Sex instruction for older people.   2. Older people—Sexual behavior.
  I. Spitzer, Cindy.   II. Title.
  HQ55.L96 2010
  613.9'60846—dc22

                                                                2009053953

Publisher: Health Communications, Inc.
         3201 S.W. 15th Street
         Deerfield Beach, FL 33442–8190

Cover design by Larissa Hise Henoch
Interior design by Lawna Patterson Oldfield
Interior formatting by Dawn Von Strolley Grove

In the musical *The King and I,*
by Richard Rogers and Oscar Hammerstein,

Anna sings:
"When you become a teacher, by your students
you'll be taught . . ."

I first heard Gertrude Lawrence sing these words
when I was young.
It took me all these years to finally understand
what they meant.

To my clients,
who have entrusted me with their souls
and have taught me so very much

CONTENTS

ACKNOWLEDGMENTS

Dorree Lynn

Sometimes stars align and one humbly and with appreciation says, "Thank you." That is the case with this book's team. They have been beyond wonderful. Talented writer and gem of a human being, Cindy Spitzer took my beginnings and endings and made the middle—actually the entire book—so much better than I could have alone. Cathy Phillips, executive assistant par excellence, kept my life functioning, while researching and endlessly proofing the manuscript. Allison Janse, our HCI editor, was continually supportive and creative. My agent, Linda Konner, made a great match getting me to HCI. And what is so wondrously special about this collaboration is that we are individuals of different ages and life stages.

My sincere appreciation goes to my friends, Dr. Fern Loos Beu, Joyce Bonnet, and Dr. Mary Liepold; to my colleagues at AARP, producers Nina Halper and David Pepper, who coined me their media "sexpert"; to my readers and supporters Sheridan Brown, John Crawford, James (Jim) Gross, Gwen Pearls, Lesley and Rick Wolfson, and Jerry Martin, my computer guru; to adult toys expert, Tamara Payton Bell; to my focus group participants who spilled their concerns and questions (perhaps all the wine helped); to my extended family "clan"; and of course, to my funny, generous, loving husband, Isaac Levy, who willingly lived with my computer love affair when I'm sure he would have preferred me in bed.

Cindy Spitzer

Thank you, Dr. Dorree, for trusting me with this fun, true, and important book. We sprang into each other's lives at just the right moment, like the ice cream truck suddenly rolling down your street on a hot summer day. I admire your guts, smarts, humor, and wisdom. It has been a pleasure and privilege collaborating with you.

I also thank my wonderful husband, Philip Terbush, precious children, Chelsea, Anya, and Zachary, and dear friend Cindi Callanan, for our shared love and support. I am also filled with gratitude for two extraordinary teachers who helped set me on the path toward the life I now love: Christine Gronkowski, who at SUNY Purchase in 1985 showed me what I could not see in myself; and my fabulous writing mentor at UMCP, two-time Pulitzer Prize–winner Jon Franklin, whom I haven't seen in more than two decades but still learn from daily.

FOREWORD

By Devra Lee Davis, Ph.D., M.P.H.

For most of her life, Dr. Dorree Lynn has been breaking paradigms. As a teacher, psychologist, and public speaker, she has paved the way to staying sane in a multi-tasking jam-packed world. In a world awash with prescription drugs and fix-it books for everything from our minds to our libidos, she brings a refreshing grown-up approach to one of the most important parts of life—our ability to reach out and touch someone and feel alive, exuberant, and connected. She exposes the myths of eternal youth and instant orgasm with élan and great wit that is both frank and captivating. Dr. Dorree shows us that the simple medical model that primarily promotes drugs to treat changing sexual performance must often be rejected. There are truly many different ways to skin a cat and many different paths to feeling intimate, passionate, and connected as we age.

For those of us who have reached the age of some distinction, advertising images provide a constant reminder that we aren't as young, as thin, or as smart as we used to be. But saying we aren't kids anymore does not mean that we are less of a person or less able to enjoy delicious moments of intense joy.

The brain remains the sexiest part of the body. If we are lucky as we age, we still remember the feelings of youth and all the drama and intensity that surrounded some of the simplest and most important parts of our relationships. But if we listen to Dr. Dorree, we will learn not to confuse those memories of what once was for what passion and love are all about as we enter and maneuver through the second half of our lives.

Thomas Moore once noted that we have a habit of talking about sex as something that is merely mechanical. Yet, nothing we do has more soul. As we age, we can find new ways to allow sex to transform us, enthrall us, center us, and calm us. To accomplish this well, we have to reject the cultural view that sees the body as detached from our feelings, our sense of values, and our emotions. Staying in love or falling in love again in midlife, or falling in love over and over again with a still lovely spouse as an elder, requires a sense of humor and a keen appreciation that hope is one of the most powerful stimulants in the world.

Dr. Dorree teaches us that our habits and expectations—no matter how well established they are—can get us into trouble and need to change as we do. As Moore explains in *The Soul of Sex*, "Sex takes us into a world of intense passion, sensual touch, exciting fantasies, many levels of meaning, and subtle emotions. It makes the imagination come alive with fantasy, reverie and memory." Accepting the constructive role of sex and play throughout our lives, as Dr. Dorree urges, helps free us of guilt and feelings of inadequacy. If we succeed in doing this, we will pay more attention to beauty, sensuality, and pleasure, and enhance our enjoyment of the full experience and our own spirituality, as well as increase the quantity and quality of fun in our lives.

This book offers much more than the usual techniques found in how-to-do-it sex cookbooks. With added years our physiology changes and for most, so does our physical desire (both more or less). While the physical expressions of intimacy can change, the need for physical, spiritual, and emotional intimacy is the one constant. Lifelong partners need to work at finding new ways to satisfy themselves that fit the changes in their bodies, minds, and souls.

Here you can find information in an easy, digestible way that manages to be both amusing and profoundly important. Many typical sex books break things down into their smallest component and miss the really big picture. As a result, the ordinary book on this topic takes the juice out of sex and is frankly boring. With a breezy style that is unafraid, Dr. Dorree presents the physical part of sex as a central component of life that cannot simply be treated or managed with drugs alone.

What works for one person may not work for another. There is no one size fits all to our private parts or our private feelings about this most essential part of life. Despite its universality, sex remains a uniquely personal experience that is tailor-made for each individual and each couple. Dr. Dorree wants people to understand the need to take responsibility to learn and grow as they explore changes in their own sexuality, their feelings and bodies that come with the privilege of growing older.

Sex for grownups provides a welcome approach to an age-old problem: how to remain vitally alive and sexy as we age. Dr. Dorree reminds us that we can start with accepting who we are and understanding that the best things in life change as we change. Expectations of that twenty-something-year-old we once were are remembered and put behind. With grace,

some technical help, abundant good humor, and a willing attitude, this book shows you how those golden years can be full
of fun and good feelings that last a lifetime.

Devra Lee Davis is the author of *The Secret History of the War on Cancer* (Basic Books, 2009*)*,
and National Book Award finalist *When Smoke Ran Like Water* (Basic Books, 2003), and *Sell
Phone: What's Really on the Line* (Dutton in 2010). She is the founder of Environmental
Health Trust and Visiting Professor of Preventive Medicine at Mt. Sinai Medical Center.

INTRODUCTION:
Yes, We Still Do It!

Welcome to the wonderful, sometimes confusing, and always exciting world of sex for those of us who (gratefully) are long past being kids. When it comes to the often discussed but rarely personally understood topic of sex after 50, mature adults tend to fall into two camps. Either you inwardly smile, knowing that grownup sex, like fine wine, just gets better and better with age, or you shrug your shoulders and say, "Sex after fifty? Does it really exist?" The truth is sex after 50 really can exist, and though it may be different from what you remember when you were younger, it can actually be even *better* than before.

If you find that hard to believe, you are not alone. As a practicing psychologist, Dr. Dorree speaks with women and men every day who find sex has become a bore, a chore, or a source of performance anxiety. Often in secret, people over 50 quietly worry about a myriad of sexual issues that are more common than most of us think.

For example, if you're a woman, do you find your mind wandering away from the bedroom? Does the thought of graying hair, a widening waistline, or sagging boobs make you

INTRODUCTION: Yes, We Still Do It!

want to undress in the closet? Do you fret about your turkey neck or secretly look in the mirror and pull your skin tight, pondering what creams or a surgeon's knife might fix?

If you're a man, do you worry about getting it up and keeping it up in bed? Or maybe you're self-conscious because your penis seems smaller and less cooperative than before. Do you wonder if any other guys think the way you do?

While it's easy to think there is something wrong with us now that we don't look like Barbie and Ken or perform like athletes in bed, in truth we are as normal as can be. It is perfectly natural for our bodies to change as we age. And of course, sex changes too—which, with some new information and a willingness to experiment, can turn out to be an unexpected gift. Just when we think we are losing something special from our youth, we have the opportunity to experience something that can be even more marvelous, now and in the future. In fact, we can remain sexually fulfilled beings as long as we are alive. Sex makes the world go round. It is our essential life force, within us through every age and every life stage. In fact, lifelong sex is what sets us apart from all other species.

However, in today's sex-flooded, youth-focused world, it's easy to find superficial sex information served up on "reality" TV (which is not at all real) or in popular magazines, but where can you go for real wisdom and practical solutions that go beyond Viagra and cosmetic surgery? As Americans, we like to think of ourselves as so sophisticated and so in-the-know about sex, but many of us really don't know where to turn for truly useful insights about what's happening to our bodies and how we can still have deeply satisfying sex at every age and stage, no matter how we change.

You are not now, nor will you ever be, too old for sex, too ill for sex, too unattractive for sex, or too alone for sex. Despite Madison Avenue, the media, and the medical world telling us that only young is sexy, the truth is that each of us can be sexy for all of our lives—far more sexy than most people imagine. While it's true that sex does change as our sex-drive hormones begin to fade after 50, our core sexuality lasts a lifetime. Sex never dies!

Sex is just too primal, pleasurable, and good for us to give up without a battle. At any age, sex can keep you healthier and may help you forget about your worldly woes for a while. After 50 (and even after 90), we don't need to toss out our condoms and hang up our vibrators as we grow older and wiser. Sex and sensuality are integral and permanent to life, and there is no reason, if we are physically able, not to enjoy both for the rest of our days.

However, it takes some new knowledge and effort, and maybe even some new ways of thinking about yourself and your partner, and that is where this book comes in. *Sex for Grownups* goes boldly where other books only peek—into the intimate lives of real adults having sex (or wanting to) in their 50s, 60s, 70s, and beyond. Whether you are a 50-year-old woman just beginning menopause or an 85-year-old man who hasn't been intimate with another person in more than ten years; whether you can't last as long as you used to or you have an illness; or you are just plain bored in the bedroom, this book is your gateway to a sexy new future. Within its pages you will find many things you may never have heard of or read before that could very well change your life. The idea is to transform your thinking and shift your attitudes. While the book is full of practical tips, information, and new things to try in and out of bed, it is by no means a technical how-to book on the pure mechanics of sex. It's a book about *morphing your mind*. What you decide to do with your body is up to you.

We hope the book helps you talk to your loved ones, partner, friends, and those who want a chance to open up more about what we all know is so true. Sex after 50 can be great, but getting there requires a bit of an attitude shift and the journey is not without some bumps. We're sure you'll find that most of what we are about to share with you about sex in the second half of life is really quite reasonable, sometimes comforting, and even funny at times.

Feel free to just dive into the chapters and sections that interest you most. Women will probably gravitate to Chapter 2 ("Sex Is More Than Procreation") and Chapter 4 ("Keeping Your Juices Flowing"). Men may want to take a look at Chapter 3 ("Performance Power Customized") and Chapter 9 ("The Great Joyride"). If your relationship is on the rocks or could just use a tune-up, Chapter 6 tells it like it really is in a long-term relationship and how to fill in those lost intimacy, fall-in-love-again gaps. Looking for a partner? Check out the many tips in Chapter 7 ("Plenty of Fish in the Sea"). Those with illnesses and physical challenges (eventually we all have something or our partners do) can turn to Chapter 8 ("Illnesses, Schmillnesses!") for new ideas about how to make love if you are no longer an acrobat. And we hope that everyone reads Chapter 1 ("You're Still Rockin'") and Chapter 5 ("Between the Sheets"), which finally set the record straight about real sex as we age and offer countless suggestions for turning so-so sex into really good sex, and making really good sex even better.

Throughout the book, the personal stories and questions are all true. Even better, the answers are, too! Psychologist Dr. Dorree Lynn has helped thousands of people over the last four decades with her healing wisdom about relationships and sex. So if you are feeling down about your lack of spark (and we all sometimes do), don't deny your sexual desires until they flicker and fade. Sex is your birthright and you deserve to be happy at every age! This book will show you how.

ONE

YOU'RE STILL ROCKIN' AND WE DON'T MEAN IN A CHAIR
Change Your Attitude, Change Your Life

Once upon time in America, there were many people approaching 50 and even more after 50, who were rapidly becoming the major age group in the land. Despite this fact, these pioneers were still trying to hang on to the youngsters they remembered themselves to be. They wanted to look younger, act younger, feel younger, and especially have sex like they did when they were younger. After all, everyone on TV and everywhere else said staying young forever was a good thing and certainly quite possible. And who doesn't like being told you can have exactly what you think you want, for as long as you want it? Who among us would dare to whisper that the Myth Emperor has no clothes; that youth fades, gravity happens, hormone levels fall, and time marches on? We are all happier with easier pleasantries and a few good myths to cling to (including, by the way, the authors of this book). How else can we live happily ever after?

Fairy tales always end with the prince and princess somehow finding each other, but you'll notice they never show what happens next. We gladly put up with the miseries of Cinderella scrubbing the floor earlier in the story because we know she will get the hunk in the end. And we're just as happy not to see what happens later, when Cinderella is back on her knees, scrubbing up baby puke and feeling abandoned by her prince. The messiness of real love, real sex, and real life are not the stuff of fairy tales. That's why Sleeping Beauty is awakened by a kiss at the *end* of the story, not at the beginning. After that kiss, all the juicy foreplay, the sticky sex, the relationship issues, financial strains, communication breakdowns, and all the other downs and ups of real life are magically missing from our fairy tales. Given how complex life actually is and how differently women and men view both the process and the goal, it's a wonder that anyone manages to have a good relationship at all.

In the real world, real men and women can still manage to feel sexy and even live happily ever after—but only *after* they challenge the myths, ignore the lies, and start exploring some new grownup must-tries that can make sex after 50 truly magical.

Why must we reconsider our beloved myths? Because the very myths that are so appealing earlier in life (the idea that we never have to grow older and sex will never change) can end up hurting us later in life when we try to cling to these myths instead of embracing our new reality. Quite naturally, none of us wants to think about getting older or possibly losing our youthful sexuality until we are forced to. Those in their 40s might still intend never to grow old, read every magazine sex article they can find, and only fleetingly wonder why they feel a bit more tired than before. In our 50s, we may begin to have concerns about new facial lines, menopause, or softer penises. In our 60s, perhaps our energies are less reliable and intercourse becomes more challenging. Each step of the way, we may feel increasingly bad about our changing bodies and maybe even feel like failures in bed when we cannot live up to our own expectations of youth. And then one day, who knows when, maybe in our 70s, 80s, or beyond, we realize that layer by layer our myths of youth are all gone and that there was no point in trying to be anything but our true selves at every age and stage. How much more amazing life could be if we realize this sooner so we can enjoy each precious moment more, rather than perhaps spending so much time chasing a lie for the sake of a dream, believing a myth that once felt so good, until it started to hurt so bad.

The truth is we do age. We grow, we change—and sex changes, too. Sex after 50 can be deliciously satisfying, but since life is not a fairy tale, we don't get to have it that way without making some effort. There is no right or wrong way to enjoy sex after 50, and we all stumble and bumble along the best we can as we travel this new road. With some new ideas along the way (maybe like some of the ones in this book) and some effort, life *can* be happily ever after—sort of. While not perfect, that's far better than any make-believe fairy tale.

Dr. Dorree Says:

When the fairy tale fades, men and women continue to have different story lines.

What a Difference a Lay Makes

Bill felt depressed. At 57, his hair was falling out and his energy was down. Worst of all, he just couldn't seem to get and keep an erection like he used to. For as long as Bill could remember, he could always count on his penis to perform. Now he worried he might be over the hill. Then

one day his wise wife made love to him, and shazzam!—a
new Super Bill emerged (for a while, at least).

A Connection a Day Keeps Sex in Play

Bill's wife Gail, 55, feels awful. She still loves her husband, but lately married life has become more bother than
fun, especially in bed. With hot flashes, cold sweats, and
droopy body parts, she'd rather just keep to herself. Who's
got the desire or energy for sex? She would much rather
cuddle and talk in bed (preferably with her sleep gear on
and the lights off), and skip intercourse altogether,
although she's willing to occasionally please her husband.

For Gail, the intimacy is mightier than the orgasm. Both
feel that something precious is slipping away as their bodies change and sexual desire wanes—and neither knows
what to do about it.

Who's That Stranger in Your Mirror?

Do you think people your age look much older than you?
Have you noticed men balding on top and widening in the
middle? Are your women friends trying to wash away their
gray and cram themselves into the hippest (and more hip-
accommodating) Not Your Daughter's Jeans?

It's hard to believe, but you've changed, too. Maybe
you're feeling a little heavier and a little slower than before.
Maybe your kids have grown, work has changed, relationships are different, and sex just isn't as much fun, exciting,
or intimate as it used to be. Or maybe you've never married
or are suddenly single and wondering what to do.

As you approach 50 and after, body fat increases, skin gets drier, energy flags, body parts sag, and your sex-drive hormones drive off into the sunset without you. Few of us are ever really prepared to age. We all know it's bound to happen "someday," but not today, and certainly not to us. It all creeps up so slowly, hardly noticeable at first. Then one day, the reflection in the mirror doesn't match the person you still feel you are inside. Your body has changed, your life has changed—*you* have changed.

Now it's time for your thinking to catch up.

Simple Stats to Start You Thinking

- 14.7 percent of Americans will be over 65 by the end of 2010, according to the U.S. Census Bureau.
- 25 percent are already over age 50.
- 40.9 percent will be over age 45 by 2010.

That means about four out of ten Americans are in the second half of life. What kind of sex are all these folks having? Does sex change, stay the same, or just fade away? What can we expect of our sexuality as we age?

The simple answer is there are no simple answers. People over 50 enjoy sex in countless different ways: with partners and alone, frisky and relaxed, often and infrequently, routine and exotic, with emotional intimacy and without it, married and unmarried, in sickness and in health. Some people over 50 do give up sex entirely, but most do not. While sex in the second half of life does change over the years, it never dies.

Can Sex Really Last a Lifetime? The Answer Is Hiding at Your Local Nursing Home

If anyone wonders whether we stay sexy and sexual for our entire lives, consider something few people know: Behind closed doors at nursing homes across the country, older adults are continuing to enjoy sex in their 70s, 80s, and beyond. That's right. Grandma Sadie and old Uncle Lou are sneaking around like teenagers, kissing, cuddling, and even more, every chance they can get, whenever that cranky young nurse turns her back. And why not? Hot, juicy love makes the world go round, and sex is an important part of the equation. For most of us, sex-drive hormones do fade with age, but our core sexuality can last forever and our sensuality can expand. Whether it's heterosexual, homosexual, bisexual, transsexual, or a banquet for one, sex is part of our deepest selves and a vital path to our primal connection with others.

Not only that, sex is good for us! In fact, studies show that people over 50 who have a regular sex partner tend to be happier, healthier, and may even live longer than those who miss out. For example, in a 2004 AARP Sexuality Study, respondents who said they had a regular sex partner generally reported having a more positive outlook on life, feeling less stressed, are less likely to be depressed, and are more likely to report their health is excellent or very good. And all the other health benefits aside, good sex is just plain fun. That alone is more than enough reason to try to keep it alive.

The challenge for those of us over 50, as we live longer than any group before, is to find ways to navigate the many physical and emotional changes of aging so that we can continue (or begin!) to enjoy sex and sensuality to the fullest.

And for those active nursing home residents, who sometimes pick up sexually transmitted diseases because they don't have easy access to condoms, let's show a little more respect. If we let teenagers sleep together in colleges, why can't older adults have a little freedom and privacy? Give them free condoms and "Do Not Disturb" signs.

The Day My Butt Fell

QUESTION: *I had just gotten out of the shower and was trying to get my contacts out. I wiped away the steam from the full-length mirror and what I saw shocked me. Exactly when did my rear end fall?*

—JUANA, 49

Your bottom didn't fall; it gradually relaxed. Gravity happens! You can lift your butt somewhat with exercises that target that area or go for a whole Brazilian cosmetic surgery tighten and reshape but that's not what's really bugging you, is it? Each of us eventually has that defining moment when we realize we are no longer young. It was happening all along, of course, but suddenly we notice.

How old is old? At 49, you are pretty old compared to a 20-year-old, but still quite young in the eyes of a 65-year-old, and practically a baby to someone who was your age when you were born. Age is relative, not only to younger and older people, but also relative to how you feel about yourself, your expectations, and your culture. You can be over the hill at 35 or still young at heart at 75. Besides your chronological age, you also have a biological age (your health status compared to others) and even perhaps a psychological age (how you feel, think, and behave, relative to others).

In some real ways, age is merely a state of mind. But there is no escaping the fact that our bodies do physically age, as well. For women, menopause (typically around 51) provides a clear signal of the "change of life" as estrogen suddenly drops, but knowing what is happening usually doesn't stop it from throwing you into an emotional and physical tailspin. For guys, the impact of gradually declining testosterone can sneak up slowly, until one day your erections seem softer and less reliable than before—rarely the most welcome wake-up call. All these changes can feel like a terrible loss, and there is no quick way around the grieving process that most of us go through when we realize that the sexuality of our youth is truly behind us.

On the very bright side, we get two huge benefits as we grow older. First, with children out of the house (unless they have boomeranged back to you), careers established, work cut back, or possibly retirement, we have more time to enjoy ourselves and our partners if we have one, and more time to go find one if we don't. Secondly, as our sex hormones naturally decline, we also have a tremendous opportunity to experience deeper, closer, more sensual sex (see Chapter 2). Having more time to focus on ourselves and a greater opportunity for sensuality are each a big bonus. Together, it's like winning the lottery twice.

Who Says Younger Is Sexier?

Just about everyone, that's who! Gazillions of messages a day try to convince us that young—and *only* young—is sexy. Sure, the media throws us a politically correct nod, showing attractive seniors supposedly shining our way though our golden years, even if a bit battered and bent. But those token gestures can hardly compete with all the TV, movies, radio, popular music, magazines, and even wrappers on gum and panty hose—all full of images of young, sexy people whom we are supposed to try to be.

Why? What is so wonderful about not growing up? What is wrong with being just who we are at every age? Our culture tells us we must hang on to youth like a life raft, and with enough makeup, Botox, and sass, we really can turn back the clock. But 50 is *not* the new 30, 50 is the new 50; 60 is *not* the new 40, 60 is the new 60! After all we've been through and fig-

Dr. Dorree Says:

A tip about age. I don't go by the numbers. I calculate my age by looking behind me at those who may be younger and saying "been there, done that," and looking ahead and saying "I'm not there yet." Calculating my age by life stage makes tons more sense than by years.

ured out over the years, 50 or 60 really can be a whole lot happier and sexier than 18, or at least we can understand ourselves better. It's part of life's developmental tasks. Unlike when we were young and trying to fit into a world we just met, after 50 we can finally, proudly, and fully be our true selves. Do we really need to look and feel twenty years younger? *Didn't we already do that?*

Yes, it would be nice to have the energy and strength we had back then. But do you really want to go back and do it all over again? The teenage acne, that nerve-wracking junior prom, starting up your young adult life, perhaps raising small children, finding a first job, or building a career—isn't it nice to be finished with some of that stuff?

Most teenagers and young adults (including maybe ourselves at an earlier time) think they invented sex. They find it inconceivable to imagine that their parents, or anyone significantly older, are "doing it." Of course, in time, it dawns on most people that this can't possibly be true; of course sex is not only for the young. But the idea can linger and confuse us, especially when it is so relentlessly reinforced nearly everywhere we turn. It's true that young people at the height of their fertility can look very sexy, but grownup, intimate, authentic sex can beat the pants off awkward, training-wheel sex most every time. Even our age looks sexy, depending on the eyes of the viewer.

It's all about attitude. It's appropriate to grieve for our necessary losses, feel sad for what is no longer, bemoan our thinning hair, and whine about our waistline, wrinkles, and warts. But you can also grab ever-changing life by the tail and enjoy the ride—even if (admittedly) you do end up a bit nauseous on some of the twists and turns. *Now* can finally be your time to see life as the adventure it's always been. Of course we've changed! That's what happens when you keep living.

> **Dr. Dorree Says:**
>
> As grownups, no one else can tell us what is right and wrong. We have to take responsibility for our own decisions, and to understand that whatever we do, the choice is our own.

Blazing Our Own Trail

QUESTION: *As a 60s flower child, I went to Woodstock with my boyfriend and years later, after a divorce or two, married the guy. I can't believe I'm this old! I'm still groovin' and having sex, but I'm not sure how I am supposed to behave now. Can I still go out dancing in my tie-dyed shirt? I don't want to stay home and knit sweaters.*

— ANITA, 58

If Grace Slick of the Jefferson Airplane could see you now, we're sure she'd tell you to rock your 58-year-old tail off if it makes you feel good! For those of us who came of age in the rockin' 50s and 60s, the idea of aging may seem as stodgy as an old rocking chair. Clearly, you are not the same as your parents' generation when they were this age. And in your tie-dyed shirt, you probably don't look like the unlined Hollywood faces that we see in the media every day. Given that people over 50 are living longer now than any group before, many of us will be sticking around longer, and therefore "doing it" longer, than any generation in history. We were once trailblazers (think civil rights, the Pill, and all the rest) and now we are trailblazers again as we enter this new, uncharted territory of sex after 50, with all too few (and often misleading) guideposts to point the way.

So if you want to dance in the rain and then run inside and make passionate love with your Woodstock husband, that's entirely up to you (as long as you don't disturb the neighbors!).

What's So Great About Getting Old?

QUESTION: *Can someone please tell me what is so great about getting old? My hair is falling out, my youthful energy is gone, and my retirement account is not performing as well as expected and, frankly, neither is my dick. Just when I thought I'd be cashing in on my "golden years," it feels like all I have is a bunch of wooden nickels.*

— GEORGE, 60

Life doesn't always go our way, finances can fail, bodies change, and having a penis that isn't doing what you want can take some getting used to. Believe it or not, your less-than-super-hard penis can be your ticket to a different kind of sex that can be even better than what you enjoyed before. (By the way, we've met some men who couldn't believe this at first and now they actually do.) With new information and some effort, you can learn to have sex in new ways, which may or may not always include intercourse. There is a lot more you can do with your magic wand than pump and hump away or deliver sperm to an egg.

Of course, you want to get back to enjoying sex again, but you aren't going back, you are going forward. The first step to a better sex life may be to change your thinking. Yes, the sexual changes that come with age can feel like a blight at times, but the fact that we get to live long enough to have some of these challenges is very much a blessing.

Smile, You're on Bonus Time!

You've probably heard "I hate getting older, but it beats the alternative" or "Aging is not for sissies." These sayings even pop up on bumper stickers in retirement communities. Try thinking this way instead: "We are lucky! We're on bonus time!"

For millions of years, women did not have to face menopause and men rarely had to deal with flagging penises and enlarging prostates for one simple reason: they didn't live this long! Up until very recently, most adults did not live past the age of 35 or 40. Even as recently as the early 1900s, the average age at the end of one's life was only 51. That means, in evolutionary terms, if you are over 50 years old, you have won the time lottery! Living this long is a lucky break of gigantic proportions.

We know your joints may ache, your vagina may be drier, and your penis may have changed. We know it isn't easy to be longevity pioneers! We may be sex pioneers, too. How will you spend your lucky bonus years? Will you spend them feeling sorry for yourself because you are no longer 14 or 34? Or will you spend your extra time learning to enjoy life with everything you've got?

And what about sex? Because our bodies and hormones are changing, we cannot spend our bonus years doing exactly what we did when we were younger. In the second half of life, we have to morph ourselves. *We have to morph sex!* No one ever told us this would happen or taught us how to do it. We can't exactly expect the younger people behind us to lead the way. They can teach us new tricks, but it's also up to us to educate and mentor them. As we age, we need to blaze our own sex-after-50 path.

Living Is Good for Your Health

Birthdays are good for you. Statistics show that people who have the most are more likely to get even more. According to the National Center for Health Statistics, boy babies at the time of birth are likely to live to about 75 and girls to about 80. But guess what? The older you are, the better your odds for living even longer. That's why at 65, life expectancy jumps to 82 for men and 85 for women. And at 85, it's 91 and 92, respectively.

Mirror, Mirror, on the Wall, Can I Still Be Sexy at All?

QUESTION: *Let's get real. I'm a single, overweight, middle-aged woman. Who's gonna want me now?*

—JULIE, 59

Ever hear the expression "Inside every older lady is a younger lady wondering what happened"? Guess what? You still are that younger lady, you just evolved to be more of yourself and along the way your body evolved, too. Each season of life is beautiful in its own way. In our youth-focused culture, concerns about body image are a major libido killer after 50, especially for women (although it certainly impacts men, too). If you don't have a partner, you may wonder how in the world you will ever attract one, and if you do have a partner, you may wonder how sexy you can be. ("Am I too old for fishnet stockings, garter belts, and stilettos?") Maybe your own daughter has said you need a facelift or a boob job, and you're wondering if she's right. Or maybe just a little liposuction? Should you color your hair or let it go gray? A little tummy tuck? Would a Wonderbra help? It can all be so confusing, even anxiety producing and depressing.

One of the advantages of going through all this at our age, rather than when we were teens, is that with the years, hopefully, have come more wisdom, smarts, and self-confidence to deal with the realities of life. Thinking positively can be helpful, but that alone may not be enough to help you change. Better to face facts and accept reality than to fight it and yourself.

Of course, it's never too late to benefit from becoming more physically active and eating good food. And if it boosts your confidence and makes you happier, you can go for some cosmetic surgery, teeth whitening, or whatever else you are moved to do. You can try a new pair of jeans with a new fangled girdle built in to deal with too much junk in the trunk. You can change your hairstyle or go for a complete makeover.

Or just try focusing on what you like about your body and

yourself. Choose clothes you feel good in and create a life that highlights your best features so you can minimize what doesn't work for you and maybe find some joy. You can also seek inside for a deeper sense of self-confidence, acceptance, and self-esteem. There really is no one right way to feel sexy as you age.

Remember, you are not alone. All of us over 50 are traveling this same path. Just like you, we are trying to cope with and adjust to our changing bodies. And just like you, we want to be desired and loved. There are plenty of people right now who would love to get to know you and even date you (see Chapter 7). Before you give up on love and sex at the tender age of 59, consider this: you could be around for another 40 years so you might as well enjoy it!

A Hairy Situation

After 50, hair tends to grow thinner and slower than before. Many men simply go bald and the world considers it sexy. For women, the situation can get a bit trickier. Thinning hair during menopause can be devastating for some women until they eventually accept their new locks or secretly start seeking remedies. Ditto for gray hair, which is easier to alter.

It's one thing to find a few gray hairs on your head (first we pull, and when there's too many to yank, we can always dye). But the day that first gray *pubic* hair shows up is almost too much for a woman to bear. We get a mirror, close the bathroom door, and start hunting for more. Damn. Are we really that old?

Worse, as our overall body hair begins to depart, it seems to travel north to our faces, especially our chins! As we've heard women say, I refuse to think of them as chin hairs; I

> ## A Hairy Situation (cont'd)
>
> prefer to think of them as stray eyebrows. A whole industry
> of products and procedures has sprouted up to cash in on
> our quest to banish our billy goat hairs, from waxing, tweez-
> ing, and chemicals, to electrolysis and vibrating razors. Even
> the most back-to-nature women who rarely shave their legs
> secretly tweeze those wire-like strays off their chinny-chin-
> chins. The confusing thing is nobody seems to know that
> everyone does it. Behind our bathroom doors, we each
> think it's our own private cross to bear.

Trick or Treat?

QUESTION: *When I come home from work, my wife is a regular
witch-on-wheels. I guess it's the menopause. I don't
know. In 27 years of marriage, the fighting has never
been this bad. Forget about it in bed—definitely nothing happening there. I'm getting depressed. At the office,
my new secretary seems really sexy. Her long, young legs,
her smooth skin, her breasts . . . well, I shouldn't even
think about it because I really do love my wife, but the
truth is I'd love to have sex with my secretary. What's
wrong with me?*

—Bob, 59

There's nothing wrong with you. It's just that no one ever
told you what to expect or what your options might be. It's
terribly difficult to feel so cut off from your partner while she
goes through this major transition. Only you can decide if you
want to act on your immediate desires and risk losing the love

of your life for the sake of a quickie. Thinking and doing are not the same things. Fantasizing can enrich your sex life. So think about it all you want, and then consider the consequences before you act. A teenager doesn't usually give himself the time to ask the question you can: how will I feel in the morning?

One option is to use this situation as an opportunity to focus in on some sorely missing information about what is happening to both of you on the home front, so you can begin to put some real intimacy and great sex back into your marriage. Your wife's menopause involves deep physical and emotional changes, but these things are not just happening to her; it's something that the two of you can share, figure out, and deal with together. This doesn't have to be a terrible loss. It can be a transition to a new life, one that can lead your marriage to even greater closeness and better, mind-blowing sex than you've ever had before.

Sounds pretty unlikely, you say? With knowledge (like what you will discover in Chapters 3 through 6) and the right attitude, this can definitely happen for you!

Listen Up, Ladies: Menopause Needn't Be Men-o-Pause

Menopause—that "change of life" when sex hormones decline and menstruation stops—does not have to kill your sex life. Sure, there are some taxing side effects that come with estrogen withdrawal, like hot flashes, cold sweats, and all the rest (which we'll help you deal with in Chapter 3), but let's not lose sight of some of the major benefits of post-reproductive life.

First, there's no more monthly bleeding, bloating, backaches, headaches, and cramps. And no more periods also means no more birth control. (If you are dating, please remember you still need condoms to block sexually transmitted disease). With the kids out of the house (if they are) and with no chance of pregnancy, this could be a great time to make a little more noise and even try a few things you didn't dare before—like maybe a few new positions, sexy costumes, or even some sex toys or pornography (see Chapter 9).

But the main benefit of getting to and through menopause is the chance to spread your womanly wings and take on life in whole new ways—even sexually. In certain social circles and European countries, post-menopausal women were once considered the only suitable teachers for horny, inexperienced young men. Not that we are suggesting it as a career move, simply pointing out that mature women need not think of themselves as old discarded cows. It's true that declining sex hormones almost always downshift our sex drive after 50. But contrary to all the ads that say we should look, dress, and behave younger, mature, post-menopausal women do not have to try to be 22 (or even 42) to be just as sexy as ever—maybe even more so.

Take Morella, for example. On a recent trip to Europe to accept an education award, the widowed 56-year-old unexpectedly found herself flirting shamelessly with an attractive bus driver in Turkey. Despite the language barrier, the two hit it off so well, they exchanged phone numbers just for fun. Throughout Morella's international tour, she kept thinking about her new admirer. When all her academic meetings were finally over, she returned to Turkey for a week of fabulous sex with a man she could hardly talk to. Now back to her normal life in New York, she describes her Turkish fling as the best of her life . . . so far.

Calling All Men with Thinning Hair and Faulty Equipment

Is your hair thinning or already gone? Are you grayer than an old goose? Do you wake up several times a night to pee? Do you see a paunchy spare tire where you once had a six-pack?

Back when you were young, you wanted to make love again and again. Now you're lucky if you can just get it up. Are you wondering what changed? More important, wouldn't you love to know how to fix it?

Guess What, Guys? You're Normal

Men lack the clear signal of menopause to announce their "change of life," but after 50, men go through some big changes, too. As the main male sex hormone testosterone begins to decline, a man's only early clue may be a slightly less firm erection. Hardly grounds for calling 911. But over time, falling levels of testosterone and other hormones, perhaps coupled with prostate or other health problems, can take you to a place you never imagined you'd have to visit, no less live in for the rest of your days, a place where your fabulous, near-instant, reliably rock-hard boners are no more.

A man's interest in sex can stay robust until his final day, but the equipment doesn't always cooperate. Nobody ever tells you about all this. Did you know, for example, that many prescription medications can interfere with your ability to get and maintain an erection? In addition, medical conditions like diabetes, high blood pressure, and even obesity can make getting it hard . . . well, hard. *This has nothing whatsoever to do with your manliness.* But as a man, it would help you to know what's going on and what can be done about it.

The good news is you have a chapter all to yourself, filled with facts and information to help you figure out exactly what's happening and how to deal with it (see Chapter 4). You know you are never going to be a kid again, but that doesn't mean you can't have truly wonderful sex, maybe even better than when you were younger—but different. And if you want to really get lucky in bed, please pay attention to what we have to say about how to help transform your special lady (or in some situations, your special guy) into the sex partner you've always wanted. (Yes, this really is possible!)

No Time for Sex

It's 11:15 PM. You have a big meeting tomorrow and hoped to get to bed earlier. Your partner is snuggled sweetly under the covers, reading. It's been a while since you've made love. Too long. He/she looks so cute by the soft bedside light. You stare at your weary eyes in the bathroom mirror as you brush your teeth and wonder, *What is the point of running around all day if we can never make love at night?* The water in the sink runs cold as you swish and spit.

A quick glance at the clock: It's 11:21 PM. You wonder, *foreplay or floss?* You really should just floss and go to sleep. Flossing is very important, you know. Doctors say it might even extend your life. You pull a waxy thread from its green plastic box, open your mouth, and begin on the top.

Of course, sex is supposed to extend your life, too, right? A quickie orgasm would be nice. Yes, but she/he hates quickies and who wants to start a fight at this hour? Last thing you need right now is a big lecture about your insensitivity (or your hypersensitivity). Besides, when was the last time a "quickie" was actually really *quick* anymore? Seems like getting it hard and keeping it hard, or getting wet enough takes forever these days. Figure at least twenty minutes there. Maybe skip the flossing?

11:26 PM. Oh, the hell with it; let's just go to sleep.

Not Everyone Over 50 Fits in the Same Sex Pot

You wouldn't lump a 2-year-old in with a 12-year-old, so why think of every age and stage after 50 as the same? A 76-year-old is not a 56-year-old. Adulthood is not a static placeholder in the center of life. We enjoy different advantages and face distinct challenges at every decade. Even when we may be too busy to notice, we are always growing into our next selves as we move through each developmental stage from birth to death.

Influential psychologists Carl Jung and Erik Erikson and others have written extensively about this. As we reach our middle years and begin to fully grasp the fact that life is not infinite, we have a choice. We can try not to think about it and perhaps desperately cling to youth, or we can purposely seek to become more aware of who we are and accept ourselves so we can feel happy and fulfilled at each stage ("shrinks" call it self-realization or self-actualization).

How does sex fit into all this? Well, you wouldn't know it from watching TV, going to the movies, or reading popular magazines, but sexuality actually evolves over the course of our lives. By now, we are all aware of what explosive young sex looks and feels like. The challenge and adventure of sex after 50 is to allow sex to evolve and change as we do. It can be all buttoned-up and possibly shut down, struggling to come out like in a TV episode of *Golden Girls*. Or *Mad Men*. Or it can be out there and in your face, like *Sex in the City, Cougartown,* and *Men of a Certain Age*. And, of course, everything in between.

Starting around age 45, as we begin to lose our physical drive to reproduce, the desire for hormone-driven sex naturally starts to decline, more for some than for others. We all know menopause is coming, but few people realize that women can spend a good ten years or more in peri- or premenopause, in which their disappearing hormones have many effects (Chapter 3). Men go through many changes, too, and may begin to find their erections are not as reliable (Chapter 4), but they often say their bigger problem is getting their previously frisky ladies to want to make love as much as they used to.

During our 50s, family changes, menopause, illnesses, body image challenges, and other issues can all take their toll on sexuality. The longer you live, the less likely it is you will die of a deadly disease, but as we age, we all live with something—heart attacks, cancers, prostate problems, penile pumps, surgery, medications for this thing and that, man boobs, urinary incontinence, arthritis, sleep apnea, obesity, diabetes. We become walking examples of why the healthcare industry is exploding. Even if you don't have some health problem yourself, chances are your partner does. How we deal with (or don't deal with) these challenges sets us up for how happy we may be as we move to the next developmental stage.

In our 60s, as many people lose strength and flexibility, and may no longer be acrobats in bed, new sexual play and positions can be fun to explore. Women may consider relationships with younger men; men may seek flings with younger women, as we see with the rapid growth of "sugar daddy" websites. Long-term sexual relationships can dry up with neglect, or can become juicer than ever. In the 70s, 80s, and beyond, sex takes more effort, and sexual relationships require a good deal of self-esteem, motivation, and skills.

Which life stages are the toughest? Esteemed actress Helen Hayes, at 73, said, "The hardest years in life are between 10 and 70." What time periods are best? Dr. Dorree's close friend, a very wise woman, at age 100 said, "Every stage was new and interesting. The only part about getting older that I didn't like was that after eighty, my body took so much longer to do things, like move where I wanted to go, than I had patience for."

Life, it turns out, is both difficult and delightful. We can take heart from a children's book that adults can learn from, called *The Velveteen Rabbit* by Margery Williams (Doubleday, 1958), in which one toy animal explains to another how being loved eventually makes you "Real."

> It doesn't happen all at once. . . . It takes a long time. That's why it doesn't happen often to people who break easily, or have sharp edges, or who have to be carefully kept. Generally, by the time you are Real, most of your hair has been loved off, and your eyes drop out and you get loose in your joints and very shabby. But these things don't matter at all, because once you are Real you can't be ugly, except to people who don't understand.

Better Thinking, Better Sex

What is the biggest sex organ? (No, not that one.) It's your brain! It really is all in your head, with a little help from the rest of the body. The brain is the biggest sex organ because what we think, feel, expect, fantasize about, say, ask, and understand all creates the conditions and attitudes that we experience as sexy (or not sexy). Skin is nice and friction is stimulating, but thinking, feeling, and attitude are what really make the difference. The head leads the body.

This is equally important for women and men to understand,

and especially relevant as we age. Relying entirely on the body to become aroused only by touching and friction, without engaging the mind, can lead to frustration and doesn't work as well with age. You can't have an orgasm without a body, but you can get there a lot faster and have a lot more fun when your brain is turned on. The mind triggers the body and vice versa.

Make Love, Not Boredom

QUESTION: *After nineteen years of marriage, I am literally bored to tears in bed. After we have sex and my husband falls asleep, I sometimes cry. I don't want to leave him, but how am I going to get through the rest of my life like this?*

—TRACY, 52

How about changing it? At 52 you could have another forty or fifty years ahead of you. You don't have to suffer like this. With a little playfulness, some new information, and a spirit of shared adventure, you and your husband can get off your ho-hum treadmill and try on some new attitude.

It's not unusual for long-term couples to fall into repeating patterns—the same meals, same conversations, same ways of arguing, same ways of making love. Break out! If you feel shy or just don't know what you might like, one place you could start is with a little solo sex first, when you have some privacy to relax and experiment. Many men masturbate regularly, with or without a partner. But some women may be more reticent in this area. At any age, experimenting alone with vibrators and sex toys can spark up a woman's energy.

Once you get your juices flowing again with masturbation,

you may want to try a few of the suggestions in this book with your partner. In time your renewed partnership, improved communication, new sexual positions, role-playing, fantasizing (together or alone), greater sensuality, moaning and groaning a little (or a lot), and other fresh experiences can make a long-term relationship feel as exciting and new as a secret affair. For some couples, pornography can also help get you both in the mood, although what turns on a man may not be all that exciting for a woman, and vice versa.

The most important thing to realize if you want a better, richer, more satisfying sex life is that no one is going to magically make it happen for you, like a kiss from a fairy tale character. Your sexual experience is literally in your own hands (and head). This is great news because it means you have the power to change it if you like. Will it take some effort? Probably. Might it also involve some courage and a little experimentation? Maybe, maybe not. This much we know for sure: the myth that only young is sexy is a lie. Sex and sensuality last a lifetime and at 52, 62, or even 92, you're still hot!

TWO

SEX IS MORE THAN PROCREATION
As Sex Hormones Wane,
Sensuality Gains

You know how at the end of a really fun party, things can start feeling a bit blue? All the lovely multicolored balloons may have begun to deflate and streamers litter the floor. Imagine if, just as you were about to go, a hidden door unexpectedly opened and you had a chance to enter a secret "after party" full of new colors you've never seen before, new tastes you've never tried, and a loving friend welcoming you to join in.

That's how sex after 50 can feel if you can open your thinking, look at sex in new ways, and allow yourself some extraordinary new experiences you may not have expected back when the first party was going strong.

Men and women experience big physical and emotional changes as our sex hormones, like party balloons and streamers, begin to fall. It may seem as if we are losing something that we *must* have in order to be attractive, have sex, or feel sexy (like reliably rock-hard erections, our girlish figures, firm skin, and so on). In truth, these lovely, transient things never were our full selves, and they are not required for us to feel and be sexy all of our years. Rather than losing something essential, we are actually *gaining* the potential for something exciting and new—a deepening sensuality that can be so much more than the sex of our youth. With age and experience, a young man's drive for sexual conquest can become a mature man's quest for sexual wisdom. And the self-confidence of an attractive young woman can evolve into a different kind of attractiveness that comes with the self-knowledge and acceptance of becoming a smart and sexy sage.

None of this, of course, changes the fact that life after 50 (just like life before 50) can sometimes be as hard as hell. Life at every stage takes work, and good sex in the second half of life may require some new learning, a little experimentation (or a lot!), and probably some effort. That's because it doesn't happen as automatically as young sex may have happened for you in the past. You may have to reach out and actively open the door to this next adventure. Society, and even our peers, often don't do much to help; you often have to make it happen on your own or with your partner. Any energy you put into expanding your thinking and learning how to experience sex in new ways may bring you more pleasure, better health, greater intimacy, and even self-discovery.

With any luck, you are going to keep getting older. Why let the party peter out when you can add more pleasure to your years?

Who's Ready for the After Party?

At 52, Cane is newly divorced and running around playing the field in ways he used to only fantasize about. "I love my new life and I'm glad I have Viagra to keep me going when I need it."

At 57, Lidia, recently remarried, is having a total reawakening experimenting with being more sexual and sensual than in her first marriage.

At 59, Milton is internally railing against turning 60. Shy and introverted, he's getting depressed and sees no partying possibilities ahead, only doom and gloom.

Sherry, 65, is dating a 49-year-old man who treats her like a queen. "Where I'm from in Hungary, it's no problem for an older woman to be with a younger man."

Kramer, 71, has decided to take a class in tantric sex with his wife of 40 years. He says they don't have intercourse as often but when they do, "it's heavenly!"

Martha, 82, who now lives in a nursing home, says, "These nurses don't understand that my imagination is not stuck in a wheelchair and they don't know whose room I go to when I sneak out at night. I'm not too old to have fun!"

There is no one way to enjoy yourself fully in the second half of life. Sex goes on, it changes, and it can last forever—or not. It's all up to you and how you think.

- Do you think there is sex after 50?
- What do you imagine after-50 sex to be?
- Do you think you have to use it or lose it?
- Is orgasm required?
- Can you enjoy sex by yourself?
- Do you think boring sex can heat up again?
- What is your version of fresh fireworks?

What Is Sex?

At this stage of the game, you probably feel you know just about all there is to know about sex. (Almost everyone we've spoken to or interviewed for this book thought they did.) But our instinct that many are puzzled was confirmed. And if you are like most people, you also possess some spotty information and maybe even a few faulty beliefs, some of which may now be preventing you from fully enjoying your evolving sexuality.

What exactly is sex? It seems like a simple enough question, but answering it may not be so simple. Many people tend to think of sex as the penetration of a vagina (or anus) by an erect penis, typically ending with one or both parties having an orgasm. While sex may involve intercourse, it can be so much more. For example, you can have oral sex, with or without orgasm, which some people say doesn't count as "real" sex. (Remember that infamous presidential line, "That depends on what your definition of 'it' is"?) What about side-by-side masturbation, in which neither party even touches the other? And then there's phone sex and Internet sex, in which the participants aren't even in the same room. Does that count as "real" sex?

To our way of thinking, sex includes all sexual arousal, sexual actions, and sexual experiences that a human being can have, alone or with others, with or without touching, with or without penetration, and with or without orgasm. Sexual kissing, caressing, touching, licking, sucking, humping, penetrating—it's all sex, even if you are alone in a dark room with your hand. The friction of bodies rubbing together, clothed or unclothed, is enough to bring sexual pleasure. And just thinking about sex, reading about sex, or looking at images of bodies or people having sex are all pathways to sexual stimulation and gratification.

Bottom line: if is feels sexy, it's sex!

Use It or Lose It

Statistics show that good sex helps keep relationships going, and good relationships help keep sex going. Still, sex, like any other physical activity or skill, takes practice. Sex is the best exercise around, with or without penetration or even orgasm. As with a consistent exercise regimen, regular sex keeps your sex organs healthy, while lack of sex reduces the blood supply to your sex organs and can eventually make them unresponsive.

Although sex can be fun and increase intimacy, if you need another reason to keep your sex life active, try a medical one. Sex benefits your hair, skin, and nails. It gets your heart pumping, supports balanced hormone production, burns calories, and helps reduce stress. Good sex can even potentially offset or prevent depression and anxiety, improve sleep, and may reduce the need for some medications. There is even some evidence that breast cancer survivors who engage in sex (either alone or with a partner) recover more quickly than those who do not. That's a lot of good reasons to consider reactivating a dull sex life or starting all over again.

Dr. Dorree Says:

Think about our chaotic world. One thing is sure: sex is recession-proof and love is depression-proof. Good sex can add to our happiness, self-esteem, and relationships at every age and stage.

If you are not in a sexual relationship, you can stay sexy and sensual by taking care of your body and feeding your senses. Walk in the woods and drink in the sight and sounds of nature. Keep cut flowers in your home or office to enjoy their fragrance and beauty. Watch pornography if you like that, or read erotic literature. Do whatever you do to keep your sensual juices flowing. Stay connected to people, even if you have no sexual contact, and don't be afraid to masturbate. Staying sexual and sensual will keep your vitality going and growing.

Sex is a way of being in the world and how you feel about yourself, not just something you do with a partner in bed. Sex is more than penetration, which is optional. Sex is more than your orgasm, which is optional. Sex is more than your partner's orgasm, which is optional. In fact, even a partner is optional!

For those of you who are more goal-driven, reading this sort of thing may make you feel like screaming, "Oh, stop it! Sex is all about intercourse and orgasm, and all the rest of this change your attitude stuff is la-la land and simply silly." Though it may be an unwelcome and even boring message, or one that you don't agree with, try to listen up. If right now you can have intercourse and orgasm, that's great. But so many people have told us—and studies confirm it—that intercourse and orgasm do not always continue, but sex absolutely can live on. Maybe you will have intercourse and orgasms for the rest of your life. Maybe you won't. What's wrong with knowing something about what could be ahead? The more we know about all our options the better.

Never Too Late!

QUESTION: *It seems like the longer my wife and I are together, the less we make love. I always wanted more sex than she did and that felt bad. But in the last year, my erections aren't what they used to be, and now she's the one who wants to make love more and I'm not so sure I can. Is it too late for us?*

—RAY, 57

It can be very frustrating when you first realize that "old faithful" (your penis) can't deliver like it used to. So what are you going to do, just give up on the party now that your wife is finally in the mood?

Many people say that as they have aged, they have evolved new ways of being sexual. Instead of the super-stud, wham-bam-thank-you-ma'am sex of their youth, they have experimented with different permutations, positions, and possibilities. For most people, the process can become slower, richer, fuller, and better than ever. But the learning curve requires us to be more vulnerable and exposed, and that can be scary. Up to this point, most of us were too busy making our lives in the present to think about how to live them in the future. The word "intimacy" may not even have been in our life lexicon. Who had time or inclination? Performance-oriented intercourse, culminating in a predictable orgasm and a quick trip to the bathroom, does not always involve deep intimacy. Talking secrets together, cuddling, touching, caressing, connecting, kissing, and allowing yourself to deeply melt into someone else, who at the same time is melting into you, is a different experience—a deeper level of intimacy that you can have for the rest of your life, even as your body and health change.

Getting from wherever you are to wherever you want to go will take some effort. But we don't think it's drudgery, do you? It's both an inner exploration and an external execution that involves other people. There's even opportunity to become more "holistic" and learn about the sexual arts from the East, such as Indian kundalini. In the last decade or so, the ancient Indian art of tantric sex has been quietly slipping into American bedrooms. Rather than the usual foreplay-intercourse-climax, tantric sex teaches lovers how to extend the peak of sexual ecstasy—sometimes for hours—so that both women and men can experience several orgasms in a single sexual encounter. (See Chapter 5 for lots of ideas for great sex from 50 to 100.)

Enjoying a New Joy Stick

After so many years of reliable pleasure, the loss of youthful erections can take some time to get used to, which is understandable (see Chapter 4). It may feel bad at first because this change is mixed in with all the other changes of aging (like less energy, less physical power, perhaps illness), and so it can feel like just one more loss. But the actual physical experience of a softer erection is really not all that bad. In fact, some guys say it actually feels *better* than before.

Here's how Walter, 57, describes it: "At first, I was depressed. I couldn't keep a hard-on for too long. I felt like a failure, an old man. It really sucked. But after a while, I noticed that the skin on my semihard penis can slip around more and that feels really, really good—maybe even better than when I was younger." Plus, he says, taking longer to come is also a benefit. "It makes me take more time in bed and that has made me try more things. My wife says it's the best sex she's ever had."

Holistic Sexuality: The Sum Is Greater Than Your Parts

When we were younger and our sex hormones were running hot and fast, sexual attraction often led to sexual arousal, and sexual arousal often led to sexual intercourse, or at least the desire for intercourse. This made perfect sense at the time. After all, whether we wanted to make babies or not, we were physically at our reproductive peaks, and from a biological point of view, young sex is firmly linked to the efficient delivery of sperm to egg. Interestingly, gay male sex tends to mimic heterosexual male reproductive sex in that one partner penetrates the other and delivers sperm.

As we age, both the physical drive and ability to deliver and receive sperm efficiently naturally decline. At first, this seem baffling to us, even depressing. Men who can no longer get it up or keep it up as long or as hard as they used to often feel inadequate or fear becoming inadequate in bed. A woman in or after menopause, who experiences less vaginal lubrication due to low estrogen and other menopausal symptoms, may feel less sexy and become less responsive to her mate. With her eggs gone and her vagina drier and possibly even smaller than before, a woman's desire for intercourse may shrink as well, or perhaps even disappear permanently. And if a couple has been together for more than a year or two, it's normal for the sexual passion to wane, even without these after-50 challenges.

But here's the good part. The older we get, the more opportunities we have for discovering that sex can be more than procreation. Intercourse is wonderful and we are not suggesting that you should or will have to give it up. But there are so many additional ways to explore and enjoy your sexuality and sensuality if you expand your thinking beyond penetration to include the rest of the body, the mind, and even the spirit.

After 50, thoughts, feelings, fantasies, attitudes, and self-image turn you on (or off) more than hormones do. That means how you view yourself and your life matters more now than ever before.

Just Not That into It

QUESTION: *Lately, I've been too tired and too irritable to have sex.
It just doesn't appeal to me anymore. I love my husband,
but I cringe at the thought of having to make love every
day. I know I shouldn't say this, but I almost wish he
had erectile dysfunction so I could get a break! Is daily
sex normal? Why is it such a chore?*

—LISA, 53

It's pretty common for two people to have different levels of
desire. Most sexually active couples over age 45 make love
anywhere from once a month to twice a day, with many aver-
aging around once a week. So wanting *and* not wanting to have
sex daily are both perfectly normal.

However, if you are tired, irritable, and hardly ever in the
mood, something more than a desire mismatch may be going
on. One possibility is that you may be unsatisfied with yourself, your current life, or partnership, and your body is letting
you know. Or low self-esteem and poor body image can affect
your feelings of self-worth and sexiness. It's also very common
for unresolved relationship issues to show up under the sheets,
as well. (Find lots more on dealing with all these challenges in
Chapters 5 and 6, plus Chapter 7 if you are single.)

The number one reason for declining sex drive in women,
usually beginning in our mid to late 40s, is declining sex hormones, including falling estrogen and testosterone, as well as
other potential hormone issues, such as low thyroid levels and
adrenal fatigue. So, even if you are still menstruating and
years away from menopause, you may very likely be experiencing a drop in your hormones that could be contributing to

your declining interest in sex (see Chapter 3).

The more questions you ask, the more you learn. Talk with friends; search the Internet (remembering that the Web is good but can be inaccurate); question your doctors; and read books. With knowledge and the right attitude, every woman can be a player in her own life. Get the news you can use to thrive at every stage.

So Boring I Could Cry

QUESTION: *My husband and I have fallen into a sex routine. First we kiss once or twice, then he rubs my breasts for about two minutes, then we touch each other's genitals until he has a firm erection (maybe another four or five minutes), then we have intercourse, missionary style, and I am back to reading my magazine in about twelve minutes (ten, if I'm lucky). It's so boring I could cry. How can we change this?*

—LAURA, 58

We almost dozed off just reading all those minutes—no wonder you're so bored in bed. There are countless ways to make love differently, but first you may have to stop counting and get more into the be-here-now experience. For those of us who fell in love with Simon and Garfunkel, remember their suggestion to slow down, stop moving too fast. It really is important to make each moment last, particularly in the bedroom.

Many men get into "efficient" sex patterns, and since it usually ends with his orgasm, he may feel basically satisfied. So it's probably up to you to fix this. If it's been a while since you enjoyed sex, masturbating can be a good place to start. Masturbation has lots of benefits for women (see Chapter 3). It's good for men, too, but they tend not to need much encouragement.

Once you know better what you like, take the lead in bed by asking for what you want (see Chapter 6). Or show him without words if you think that will get your new message across. Slower sex can be very passionate if you let your energies gradually build. You might also learn a thing or two that you didn't know before, like how good his skin feels under your hands or that you like being kissed on the back of the neck.

All this added closeness can take some getting used to. It may bring some unsettled feelings, memories, and issues to the surface, giving you a chance to deal with any passion inhibitors from your past. So try getting off the clock. You just might have the time of your life!

The Gift of the Big O

An orgasm is truly one of life's most delicious gifts, one that keeps on giving with many physical, emotional, and relationship benefits. Over the years, as with most body functions, "coming" can take a bit longer to come.

What exactly is an orgasm? From strictly a medical point of view, an orgasm is the end point of the plateau phase of the sexual response cycle, characterized by an intense sensation of pleasure. For both males and females, orgasm is controlled by the involuntary, autonomic nervous system, and involves quick-cycle muscle contractions in the lower pelvic muscles, which surround the primary sexual organs and the anus. Interestingly, these muscle contractions are nearly

Dr. Dorree Says:

In this age of medical experts, the ultimate expert on you is you.

identical in both men and women, with the first few intense contractions coming at about 0.8-second intervals. As orgasm continues, the contractions become shorter and less frequent.

Some woman can experience long-lasting (a minute or longer) or multiple orgasms, which are less common (but possible) for men. Men at midlife may experience fewer or less intense contractions than when they were younger, but these are not necessarily less pleasurable. An orgasm can also involve other involuntary muscle contractions, including spasms in various areas of the body or a feeling of total body release. Some people have silent orgasms, while others flail, arch their backs dramatically, make noises, or call out words ranging from street slang to invocations of God. Some people scream loudly enough to alarm the neighbors and their partners have been known to stuff a pillow into their mouths at just the right moment.

The Truth About Blue Balls

Remember when we were kids and we joked about "blue balls?" That's exactly what happens to men. The scrotum turns a shade of blue when the blood (which is blue before exposed to air) flows into the penis and surrounding areas without the opportunity to flow out (no orgasm), leaving men with the desire to "drain their veins." Women's clitoral and vulva areas can turn a bit blue, too, although back when we were kids, few paid attention to what was less obvious. That's always been easier to do because men's sexual plumbing is mostly on the outside, while women's sex organs are mostly inside.

Orgasm in both sexes is all about blood flow, engorgement, and release. In men, chambers inside the penis fill with blood, creating an erection. During orgasm, muscle contractions propel sperm out of the penis and release the engorged blood back into the body until the erection is gone. For women, a much larger amount of blood must engorge the pelvis before orgasm (one of the reasons it can take longer for women to "come"). The

Dr. Dorree Says:

If you feel stuck in a sex rut, slow down and see what happens. One good experience can lead to another.

contractions of orgasm disburse the engorged blood, creating a wonderful sensation deep inside a woman's body. Men also have some general pelvic blood engorgement, beyond the penis itself, but the penis is usually their focal point. (See chapters 3 and 4 for more details about women's and men's sexuality.)

For both men and women, an orgasm can be a great sexual finale, providing physical, hormonal, and emotional release, and some people can learn how to have more than one during a sexual encounter. But even without orgasm, your sexual experience can be intensely pleasurable and satisfying.

What If My Husband Can't Come?

QUESTION: *My husband and I are very much in love and cherish spending time together, but he recently had surgery for testicular cancer and can no longer ejaculate. We still touch each other sexually, and I often have an orgasm when we do. Are we still having sex?*

—LOTTIE, 51

Sex is not a score card that you have to check off in order to qualify. If you both feel sensual and sexy together, even if neither of you ever had an orgasm again, it would still be sex. Sex is a

Dr. Dorree Says:

If you are not in a monogamous relationship, practice
calling your bed partner an
endearing term rather than
a specific name. That way
when you let abandonment
fly, those heart palpitations
can be fun and not panic
about whose name you
might accidently call out!

state of mind. If you are aroused, or if
you are enjoying someone else being
aroused, you are having sex. Orgasm
is a wonderful plus if you can have
one—and we're so glad you do. But if
you can't, you can still have sex all you
want as long as you feel turned on.

There are two schools of thought
on the role of orgasm for couples. One
group of sex educators, researchers,
and therapists say orgasm is essential to maintain the sex bond between
partners. The other group says orgasm is nice but not necessary for a satisfying sexual relationship, especially if you learn
to have deeply sensual sex.

Think of it this way. When you were young, maybe you
drank beer or cheap wine or whatever else you could chugalug,
regardless of how you might feel the next day. Now you've
learned to stick to a good bottle of wine or great cognac, savor
your drink, and appreciate its subtleties as you slowly taste its
many layers that slip sensuously around in your mouth and
down your throat. Sometimes, slow sensuality can be even better than a quick bang.

When Desire Expires

Sometimes sex is the last thing on your mind. It's normal
for sexual desire to wax and wane, and even to disappear
entirely for a while. According to a 1994 landmark study of
sexuality in America conducted by University of Chicago
researchers, 33 percent of women and 16 percent of men

reported they had gone through periods of several months with no interest in sex. A Harvard University report says diminished sex drive is the most common and most elusive sexual dysfunction, and that it often exists along with one or more other sexual problems. For example, painful intercourse will make a woman less in the mood for that kind of sex play.

The same study found that 13 percent of older women who called themselves sexually active had not had an orgasm during the month before the survey, whether they had intercourse or not. If we look at that study from the prism of our "bonus years," that means 87 percent did. Pretty cool. Or in today's youth-culture vernacular, isn't the current in term "hot"?

Deciding if you have low libido is entirely subjective as there are no physical signs to measure. So what you think of as low libido may be just fine for someone else. Harvard defines low libido as "the absence of sexual fantasies or a lack of desire for sexual activity that causes personal distress." They admit that female desire has been historically misunderstood because libido does not always manifest itself in the same way in women as in men. In general, a man's desire may be driven by the goal of intercourse and orgasm, while women's desire tends to be driven by a need for intimacy, as well as by physical arousal.

Both men and women find that sexual desire flags a bit with age, falling hormones, illness, stress, and many other factors (see Chapters 3, 4, and 8). If you want more desire fire, there are many sexy ways to stoke the flames (see Chapters 5, 6, and 9).

Dr. Dorree Says:

An orgasm is greater than the sum of its parts. It floods the body and brain with feel-good neurotransmitters and can bring well-being and healing.

Who's in Control?

Sex is often personified as an aggressive male Don Juan type or as a female dominatrix with a more passive partner who's not quite as interested. So who do you think is more in control?

A surprising answer: The person with the least desire almost always has the most control. Just think about it. The one who wants it less gets to decide when sex happens. You may think this is the woman, but that's not always the case. If it is the woman, she may make having intercourse so infrequent or unlikely that a man may develop premature ejaculation.

> **Dr. Dorree Says:**
>
> Orgasms are wonderful, but kissing, cuddling, touching, and saying "I love you" are all part of sex, too.

He feels he's entered a slightly opened door that may just as quickly close. Better get in and out as quickly as possible (his penis thinks). On the other hand, if it is the guy who controls sex because he wants it less often, the woman may become insecure, bitter, angry or whiny. She's ready for fun and he's got no loaded gun.

Lonely Together

What do you call a couple who has become so familiar with each other, so worn out with all the doings of life, so jaded in their relationship, and so bored in their routines that by the time they go out to dinner they may find themselves sitting at a restaurant table, together but lonely, grunting that another table might be more appealing, or perhaps secretly fantasizing about someone else who may or may not be present?

You'd be surprised by how many people answer "married."

Of course, not all long-term relationships are this dreary. (If you've lost the art of intimacy, see Chapter 6.)

Fresh Fireworks

Do you remember your best kiss ever? Maybe it was your first kiss, or your first kiss with your first true love, or your last kiss with your current mate. Do you remember petting in the car or some other uncomfortable place that at the time felt like heaven on earth? Do you remember the quick, breathless excitement, or the slow, gentle touches? Those were magical moments of connection with another person that we may remember for a lifetime.

Do you still have those special sparks that turn you on or make you feel cherished and oh-so-close with your partner? Do you stroke his/her hair as you pass their chair, or whisper sweet nothings before falling asleep? Or have years of marriage and the daily grind of life worn you down to the point where you barely remember to offer a perfunctory kiss and hardly have the time, energy, or desire for intercourse at the end of the day, just one more mandatory item to check off on your endless to-do list? Unless you invest the time, effort, and actions to stay deeply connected with your partner, in time passion fades.

It happened to Ming and Samuel. Married for twenty-two years and at one time very much in love, the daily drain of managing two careers, raising three active boys, and now caring for Sam's elderly parents had left the couple exhausted by bedtime, only able to manage an occasional "quickie" maybe once a month, if that. Sam often complained about wanting more sex, but Ming, 54, and deep in menopause, had little interest. After sharing most of her adult life with her husband, their unsatisfying sex life left her thinking of him more as a bother than a lover. *Is it time to leave?* Ming wondered.

Dr. Dorree helped her bring her secret questions into the open, and as Ming weighed the pros and cons of leaving, she realized that she was simply in a normal relationship funk and she could talk out her issues, first to Dr. Dorree and then with her husband. It turned out that the love that had been there all along began to rekindle. Ming also temporarily went on an antidepressant to help lift her spirits as she and Sam began to talk about their experiences and reconnect.

Quitting a relationship is always an option at any age, but the older you get, the better your odds of staying together if you can identify and rectify the main issues between you. Investing time and energy in rebuilding closeness can do more than save your marriage; it can save your life. Statistics show that both men and women do better together than apart. If you've lost intimacy and connection with your partner, the "bonus years"—after you've perhaps raised a family, built your career, and weathered the countless challenges of adult life—could be a good time to pay more attention to your partner, reprioritize your relationship, and take one step at a time to improve your sex life.

Ming decided to give it a try. "I just couldn't stand the thought of starting over with someone new. I'm glad I tried. The alternative now seems so exhausting!"

Sex Without Intercourse

QUESTION: *I had cancer surgery and will probably never have intercourse again. Now what?*

—LEO, 53

For many people in your situation, it may seem like your sex life is over, but at 53, you don't have to go through the next three, four, or even five decades without sex. Maybe you can't change your anatomy, but you can change your thinking and actions.

Sex without intercourse and orgasm may seem fundamentally inadequate to many people. Without intercourse, most men tend to think it's not real sex. And if only the man has an orgasm, many women may tend to feel used. But neither is necessarily true. Anything that involves sexual stimulation and arousal is sex, including hand jobs, oral sex, humping your partner without penetration, and of course, touching of all sorts.

After you've had some time to grieve and adjust, let the experimenting and learning begin. If you don't have a partner right now, don't assume you never will. Plenty of women (and men) can find you attractive and even exciting in bed. Who knows, with all those new tricks you will learn, you could be the best lover they ever had.

A Sexless Marriage

QUESTION: *Can you really revive a marriage that is DOA in the bedroom? I just don't like sex anymore and I don't care if I ever do it again.*

—RAYANNE, 71

Dr. Dorree Says:

There are times when you want to leave. Staying and changing the relationship or starting over again may both be challenging. So think twice before you decide—either way.

If you want to give up sex forever, that's your business, but before you do, how about giving it one more try, just to be sure? Reviving sex, even if you've let it go for years, could make you both happier, healthier, and perhaps even live longer, not to mention feel closer to your husband and more fulfilled in your marriage.

Could it be that not having sex has become a long-standing habit that you don't know how to break? If so, there are some paths back to your sexier self. If you were in the habit of being passive in bed and experienced sex as something "done to you" rather than shared, then you may benefit greatly from a little self-directed relearning. If you haven't had an orgasm or any sexual experience in quite a while, you can go online and discretely order yourself a vibrator if you don't already have one. These have become as common as shampoo and toothpaste in most women's homes. Masturbate frequently and learn what you like.

Next comes the fun part—shocking the pants off your husband. If you've been sexless for a while, imagine his surprise when he finds you in bed one night without your usual nightgown or whatever you typically sleep in. For fun, you can try on something sexy or silky, or maybe nothing at all. We only wish we could be there to see his face (and then leave immediately, of course). If surprises are not his thing (or yours), try talking it over first and tell him what you want to do. Either way, take it slow and see where it goes. There's no rush. Reintroduce your bodies to each other gradually, perhaps over several days. This could be a wonderful and exciting experience, especially if you still love this man. Keep your expectations low and just give it a gentle try.

Does any of this excite you even just a little bit? At any time, you can always go back to a sexless marriage, although somehow we doubt that you will!

What If I Don't Have a Partner?

QUESTION: *I have been living alone since my wife died eight years ago. Where am I going to find someone to touch an old man?*

—JACKSON, 75

Who are you calling an old man!? At 75, you could have a good ten to twenty-five bonus years left. Even if you aren't interested in finding a new partner (please see Chapter 7 if you are), you certainly don't want to give up being touched for what could be the next quarter of a century, do you?

More touch makes you feel more alive. Many older people don't get enough touch to sustain their good health. Studies show that lack of touch makes infants more vulnerable to depression and can even erase the will to survive to the point where they become ill and even die. Even without an intimate partner, there are multiple ways to get more touch into your life. These are no substitute for full-body, loving contact but are definitely worth considering while you decide if you want to look for another mate. Here are some ideas:

- Get full-body massages regularly, from either a man or a woman. Doing so can be healing and change the way you feel about yourself. Therapeutic massage can improve your immune system function, make you feel more relaxed, and significantly decrease pain and stiffness.
- Try other types of therapeutic bodywork, such as Feldenkrais, Trager, and others. Each has healing components that work on different aspects of the body. Some of these may be covered by your health insurance. It's worth finding out.
- Give yourself daily massages, either sexual or not. It just feels good.

- Get a manicure or pedicure every once in a while, and regular hair care. These can be safe and inexpensive forms of touch, especially getting your hair washed by someone else. Don't have any hair? Ask for a scalp treatment that includes a head and shoulder massage, or even a facial. Men do that sometimes.
- Join a ballroom dance class or other dance group, or participate in other social experiences that involve movement and appropriate touch. Aside from the touch benefit, it's also good exercise.
- Get involved in doing something for someone in your community. Touching others with your heart, as well as hands, may do you both a world of good.
- Get a pet, preferably something soft and silky. Studies show that people who take care of a dog or cat tend to live longer than pet-free people. Pets can be warm and cuddly, plus their unconditional love and acceptance is uplifting, especially for loners. Plus, if you take your pet out for walks or carry them with you, they can make great conversation starters with prospective dates!

As Cole Porter schooled us: "Birds do it, bees do it; even educated fleas do it." And so can you.

THREE

FEMALE MENOPAUSE AND SEX FOREVER
Keeping Your Juices Flowing

"Can I get those groceries for you, Ma'am?" the young man asked politely. "I'm sure someone your age could use the help."

"Thank you, I'm fine," Felicia smiled stiffly and darted off to her car, tears running down the smooth cheeks of the former University of Michigan beauty pageant queen. *When did I get so old?* Young men's heads used to turn when she walked into a room. Now all they see is an old lady who needs help with her bags.

Felicia knew her husband still found her sexy, but as someone whose physical beauty used to open countless doors, her changing 62-year-old body had become a daily anti-aging battleground. Felicia poured over tons of "after-50" articles and books on how to dress, apply makeup, fix her hair, hydrate her skin, exercise, flirt, and "look younger at any age" (yeah, right!), but nothing she did could really hold back the natural changes that inevitably come with time and gravity. Always a natural girl, she really didn't believe in cosmetic tweaking or going through surgery like some of her friends, so her breasts sagged and lines were deepening around her eyes and mouth. Even six years after menopause, she still endured the occasional hot flash, too many sleepless nights, and moods shifts as unpredictable as an ocean rip tide. Her once-thick hair was thinner now and grayer, her hour-glass shape looked more like a coffee mug, and every year she felt a little slower than before.

"I knew everyone eventually ages and changes," Felicia wrote in her journal that night. "I still feel beautiful. It hurts to realize that the world doesn't necessarily see me as I see myself. I just never really thought aging would happen to me. I hate it!"

Menopause: Like Falling Off a Cliff

Unlike men, who experience such a gradual decline in sex hormones after 50 that they may not even notice it for several years, when a women suddenly runs out of eggs and permanently stops menstruating, her sex hormones nearly fall off a cliff. No matter how much you may know menopause will happen someday, many women are taken by surprise by just how challenging it can be, how deep the changes go, and how long some symptoms can last. What is it about menopause that can so rock a woman's world, why is it so confusing, and what can be done about it? There are few easy answers.

Here's what we do know. Menopause is defined as the twelve months after a woman's ovaries run out of eggs, typically beginning around age 51. Each of us is born with a set number of eggs and when they're gone, they're gone. Empty ovaries produce dramatically less of the female sex hormone estrogen, bringing on menopause. (Surgical removal of the ovaries also brings on instant menopause at any age.) Estrogen is what magically made you a girl instead of a boy inside your mother's womb. Since then, estrogen not only helped grow and shape your breasts and hips, it also helped shape your thinking, feelings, and behavior—along with countless other biochemicals that together help make you tick. So when estrogen suddenly drops, instead of tick, you may feel like you go tock!

Do You Feel Loopy, Lousy, or Lost?

Are you dressing in layers in case a hot flash forces you to strip in public? Is your vagina dry, your feet cold, or your moods cranky? Welcome to menopause! For many women, the abrupt drop in estrogen production can seem to throw the whole body/mind system for a loop. Symptoms of menopause are legendary, but few people know what is actually going on. For example, the well-known "hot flashes" of menopause (sudden flushes of intense heat around a woman's neck, face, and upper torso) are actually caused by the body going through the equivalent of a nasty case of drug withdrawal. Every primary symptom of menopause has a biologically based reason, although once you have some of these unpleasant symptoms, they often have emotional impacts, as well.

In addition to hot flashes and night sweats, declining estrogen before, during, and after menopause can also cause:

- Weight gain, especially around the waist
- Irritability
- Head and body hair loss
- Sleep disturbances

- Depression or anxiety
- Fatigue
- Mood swings
- Dry skin
- Deepening lines above the upper lip and around the mouth
- Loss of bone density
- Increased risk of heart disease and other illnesses
- Slower metabolism
- Inability to drink as much alcohol as before without hangover
- Headaches
- Difficulty concentrating
- Memory challenges
- Light-headedness
- Heart palpitations
- Incontinence
- Digestive difficulties
- Tingling extremities
- Vaginal dryness, atrophy, and/or thinning of vaginal walls
- Loss of breast firmness
- Decreased nipple sensitivity
- Loss of sexual desire
- Painful intercourse

Not exactly a great recipe for feeling vibrantly healthy, self-confident, and super sexy! It's rare to have all of these symptoms, but even two or three of the above symptoms can make life pretty miserable and enjoyable sex less likely.

Before you throw down this book and run out for cosmetic whatever-you-can-get surgery, there is a brighter side to all this doom and gloom. Believe it or not, menopause does not ring the final bell on sex and sensuality for mature women, and it can even have some silver-lining benefits. For millennia, women rarely lived long enough to experience menopause, sometimes dying in childbirth or often by the time their kids were grown. Today, a woman in menopause may still have another good half century of life coming her way. If you are among the women who must tread the more challenging path through menopause and beyond (unlike the lucky few who sail through unfazed), take heart: life, love, joy, adventure, self-discovery—and even delicious sex and luscious sensuality—can be yours around this challenging corner.

What's Happening to Me?

QUESTION: *I'm 49, the mother of four children under the age of 12, and still menstruating. Why do I feel so irritable, tired, and sometimes even shaky inside?*

—MARTHA, 49

Maybe those four kids under 12 might have a little something to do with it? Or it could be any one of a number of possibilities, including the likely chance that you are in what is called pre- or perimenopause, in which some menopause-like symptoms may start ramping up as early as two to ten years before you stop menstruating. Be aware that not all medical tests tell the full truth. Sometimes ordinary blood tests fool women (and their doctors) into not believing what they feel is happening to their changing hormones.

Of course, you may also be among the fortunate group of women who will approach and pass right through menopause with hardly any symptoms at all. These lucky ladies are in the minority in the United States, although in other parts of the world, women routinely go through menopause symptom-free, most likely due to their phytoestrogen-rich diets of fish, seaweed, and soy. (Phytoestrogens are like dietary estrogens because they are naturally occurring non-steroidal plant compounds that are chemically similar to the estrogen compound, estradiol.) Japanese women, for example, who traditionally ate many phytoestrogen-rich foods, rarely experienced any menopause effects until after they adopted a more Western diet and lifestyle.

The symptoms you are describing deserve further investigation, perhaps starting with a full physical examination by your healthcare provider. You can also take a look at the next section for ideas about hormone tests you can explore. Women's health issues are often complex, but answers can be found. And good luck with all those kids!

Is It My Hormones?

QUESTION: *One day I'm happy and relaxed, the next day I'm biting my husband's head off. I stopped menstruating four years ago and thought I was past the worst of it when my hot flashes finally stopped last year. Am I losing my mind or is it my hormones?*

—RUTH, 54

Three years of miserable hot flashes should be enough for any woman to bear, but surprisingly, menopause symptoms due to declining or imbalanced hormones can last a very long time—even decades!

You may want to ask your healthcare provider to check not only your levels of the sex hormones estrogen, progesterone, and testosterone, but also your thyroid hormone levels (T3, T4, and TSH) and some of the important adrenal hormones (including cortisol, aldosterone, and DHEA). It may be helpful to test for DHEA and other adrenal hormones because after your ovaries quit producing significant estrogen, typically your adrenal glands attempt to pick up the slack by producing more adrenal hormones (there are 150 in all) and converting some of them to estrogen and progesterone. This puts an added burden on the adrenal glands just at a time when you may already be stressed by the physical and emotional changes of menopause. (The extra adrenal output of cortisol, by the way, contributes to the added fat women tend to gain around the belly during and after menopause). After a while, the adrenals may become fatigued, possibly even exhausted, and adrenal hormones may also decline.

Standard blood and urine tests are not always as useful for determining every type of hormone. For some hormones (like cortisol), saliva tests, which assess various hormone concentrations up to four times in a day, may tell you more. But don't expect a standard gynecologist or your internist to necessarily offer you a saliva test or perhaps even know what you are talking about if you ask for one. It often takes some detective work to learn about how to test for hormones and what the results mean. You may need a cutting-edge expert well-versed in the

Dr. Dorree Says:

Menopause is complicated. If you're on a mission to better understand and affect your own complex health, you must take charge of your education and maybe even help educate your healthcare providers, as well.

latest research and alternative options in this specialty (and they may or may not be covered by insurance; always ask ahead), plus dogged persistence to explore your many options for both testing and treating hormonal issues. The quest can be exhausting and frustrating, but well worth it. Talk to friends, read books, try the Internet (cautiously), and get copies of all your medical tests to keep on file at home. Other tests to consider at your age include yearly mammograms and pelvic exams, a colonoscopy, and a bone scan.

Are you getting tired (and wondering where the money will come from) just reading about it all? There's a lot to do to keep up with your changing body, but since we are fortunate to live in a time and place where such diagnostic tests are available, we might as well take advantage of them. Looking after your health can sometimes seem like a part-time job that costs you tons of money and requires time and effort that can feel overwhelming, but remember, the life—and perhaps the marriage—you save may be your own.

A Great Guy to Have in Your Corner

Chuck, 46, had been attending Dr. Dorree's group therapy for years. Most of the members were "old geezers" who often complained about being in menopause or living with a seemingly maniacal partner in menopause. Chuck heard everything from women's stories of hot flashes and uncaring husbands to how lousy it was to be alone. From the men, he listened to how it felt to love menopausal women who no longer wanted to have sex and how appealing younger women and affairs now seemed. Many times Chuck often wanted to quit the group or at least try to steer the conversation to something that interested him, such as his kid's baseball games or his latest career venture.

Then one day, a lightbulb went off for Chuck when he realized that his wife was recently acting a lot like the women the older group members had described. Could she possibly be in menopause? She was yelling at the kids a lot, had no patience now for things that didn't used to bother her, and her libido was all but gone. Something definitely was happening.

Chuck's wife, Tara, refused to see a doctor because she insisted that at age 41 she couldn't possibly be in menopause. He convinced her to come see Dr. Dorree instead, to "work on family dynamics." In a private individual session with Tara, Dr. Dorree explained how menopause can sometimes happen early and could very well account for her sudden personality change. When Tara resisted, Dr. Dorree tried another tack: left untreated, low estrogen can dry out your skin, thin your hair, increase your facial lines, especially those around your mouth, and make your vagina pucker up—kind of like aging overnight. That got Tara's attention. She called her gynecologist, got some tests, and sure enough, her estrogen level had significantly dropped.

At first, Tara was angry. "I don't want to deal with taking hormones," she protested. But when she thought about losing her sexiness and good looks, she decided to give an estrogen patch a try. She also began exploring

A Great Guy to Have in Your Corner (cont'd)

other alternatives, like joining a gym and getting acupuncture treatments. "Thank God I had a great guy in my corner." Tara finally realized this once her hormones began to stabilize. Chuck was grateful, too, for having unwittingly picked up a world of education in his "geezers" group.

The Riddle of Hormone Replacement Therapy (HRT)

QUESTION: *I know you can't really answer this for me, but should I take HRT, like my gynecologist wants me to? My menopause symptoms are pretty severe and I'm afraid of bone loss, which runs in my family, but I'm also leery of the possible side effects of HRT. And I don't like the idea of taking any drug for so long.*

—MAYA, 56

Even your doctor can't tell you whether or not to use hormone replacement therapy (HRT). It's a complicated decision. No one knows all the answers and only you can decide what to do about taking hormones, or anything else.

Please educate yourself. There are lots of options to consider. There are actually three kinds of estrogens, plus seven kinds of androgens (including testosterone), which some women may need more of (yes, women make some testosterone, just like men make some estrogen). Research shows that as many as three-quarters of women with low sex desire may have serious androgen shortages, in addition to low estrogen. In addition to checking testosterone levels, many women benefit from testing for (and boosting with oral supplements) their low levels of adrenal hormone DHEA.

The long-term risks and benefits of HRT are largely unknown, and the research so far is confusing and inconclusive. For some people, HRT (typically with estrogen and progesterone) reduces the risks of osteoporosis and heart disease, while for others it increases the risks for breast cancer, liver problems, heart attacks, and other health issues. Most mainstream doctors say HRT with estrogen is only effective when taken within the first five years after your last month of menstruation. Other practitioners say low-dose supplemental hormones, including estrogen and others, may be helpful no matter what your age after menopause. Regardless of when you use HRT, all medications have some risk of side effects, both immediate and long-term.

If you choose HRT, your decision making is hardly over. There are patches, pills, vaginal suppositories, gels, and skin creams. Prescription medications may be synthetic or "bio-identical." Some women prefer bio-identical hormones, sometimes custom mixed by a compounding pharmacy, because they are biochemically identical to the estrogen and progesterone that your body already makes. But that doesn't mean they are risk-free. All medications carry risks, although bio-identical hormones are believed to produce fewer side effects than synthetic hormones.

If you still have your uterus and you take estrogen, progesterone will be prescribed as well. This, too, comes in many different forms and delivery methods. Testosterone, if you need it, is frequently supplied as a cream or gel that you apply to your genitalia or your skin.

But the story doesn't end there. Even after you decide what you want to try, and perhaps experiment with different hormone replacement medications until you find what works best for you, you are not done figuring it out, because over time, you are always changing. So if you go on HRT or other treatment approaches, you will most likely have to revisit these decisions, again and again, as you age.

Confusing, isn't it? There simply is no easy way to answer the HRT riddle. It takes much research and contemplation. And if you haven't already left the building to drown your puzzlement in a bowl of mocha chocolate chip ice cream, here's one more question to think about....

What About Alternative Approaches?

In the last several years, Americans have become increasingly open to alternative health care, including alternative treatments for the symptoms and health effects of menopause. While mainstream medications are hardly risk-free, more natural or alternative approaches are not entirely without risk either. For example, non-prescription natural hormone supplements, perhaps made with soy or wild yam, are generally not regulated or rigorously tested, so no one really knows if they actually work as advertised. Some recent evidence suggests that some soy components may potentially stimulate breast tumors, so "natural" doesn't always equal "safe."

As we keep saying, there are no easy answers and no one rule. In general, it may be less risky to try an alternative approach, which may or may not be effective for you. And even if you find something that works for you now, keep in mind that you may need to change your treatment approach in the future.

Some of the more popular alternative approaches to menopause include:

- Herbal supplements that act somewhat like estrogen in the body (like black cohosh and others) or can be converted in the body to progesterone (wild yam cream).
- Nutritional supplements, such as DHEA, a precursor that the body can convert into various sex hormones as needed.
- Acupuncture for easing menopausal symptoms and balancing hormone production.
- Homeopathy, which can also support the body's own efforts to reach a new equilibrium after sex hormones naturally decline.
- Exercise to boost general stamina and maximize the effectiveness of the hormones you already make (or take).
- Improved diet to build overall health and supply the nutrients needed for maximum hormone production.
- Yoga, meditation, martial arts, and other practices that help you cope better with physical and emotional stress and may even help you produce more of those pesky hormones on your own.

Dizzying, isn't it? You could spend the rest of your life learning about and trying various health approaches, if you were so inclined. The best advice we can give you is to educate yourself all you can and then do what feels right to you at the time, while being open to changing your approach in the future.

Surprise! The "Big Change of Life" May Change You

Menopause can change you in ways beyond the physical body. For some women, this change can include wanting a close relationship after years of being independent. For others, it may mean putting oneself first after years of taking care of others.

QUESTION: *For most of my life, I've known what I wanted and I set out to get it. I'm not the kind of gal who sits around feeling sorry for herself. I make things happen. I have a megacareer that I'm proud of, but lately I've been feeling empty and alone. I wasn't expecting to feel like this, and it's not something I can solve with a five-year plan and a Rolodex full of great business contacts. What has come over me?*

—Michelle, 61

Menopause can throw you for a loop, just when you think your life is on the right track.

Many women experience more than a physical change after they stop menstruating. Just as a flood of estrogen at puberty did more than just help you grow breasts and shape your body (it helped shape your brain and behavior), the loss of estrogen at midlife also can have a wide range of effects beyond the purely physical. Falling estrogen can also impact your thoughts, feelings, relationships, even your sense of identity. You are fundamentally changing, perhaps even becoming a different "you."

The changes of menopause impact each woman differently. A care-taking, family-focused woman may become more independent and self-nurturing. Or a high-powered, independent woman may for the first time seek the shelter of a loving relationship in which she can be more dependent and nurturing to someone else.

For example, after menopause, Rena, a stay-at-home mother and wife of 25 years, decided to spread her wings in new directions and get a new job (and a new man). Tamera, a working woman decided to take up painting and to travel without her husband for a while. And Rachael, a high-powered career woman who had spent many years building a life and then began to see her super success as superficial, suddenly woke up and said, "Oh, my, I forgot to have a relationship!"

It's the rare woman who is excited or happy about getting older. Menopause signals that youth is behind us, and it's easy to feel increasingly insecure as you age. When you lose your youth, you often feel as if you are losing your power and yourself. You may not feel as sexy; you may not act as sexy; and you may feel a bit depressed or anxious (those heart palpitations are mighty confusing for both you and your doctor). Feelings of emptiness may be a clue. If you are in a long-term marriage or life partnership, this may be a time to reevaluate and develop a new type of bond. Or, as with you, Rachel, rather than trying to fill your loneliness with more business as usual, you could take a chance on love and commit to a partner, someone who can share your life during the day and keep you warm, connected, and feeling secure at night. It's a big world. There are probably hundreds, even thousands, of great guys who might fit the bill. And that's where years of great Rolodex building might come in handy. What's wrong with telling a few trusted contacts that you are open to meeting someone special? Maybe it's not your usual business style, but so what? Even as a successful businesswoman, you are still busy becoming a new you. (For more ideas about where and how to find your mate, see Chapter 7.)

Running on Empty? Fill 'Er Up!

QUESTION: *I've been a giver all my life. I took care of my two little sisters when my mother was dying. I helped my husband get through medical school and then raised our three kids. Now my elderly father lives with us (can't bear the idea of a nursing home), and my husband was just diagnosed with depression. I used to love taking care of people, now it just drains me. By midafternoon, I'm beat. Short of running away from home, which is tempting, what can I do?*

—MAXINE, 59

You sound like a very lovely (and tired) person. Where are the interests and activities that feed your soul? Even the greatest chef in the world has to take some time to eat for herself. This requires feeding yourself first and learning to say no to having everyone depend on you. As your estrogen dropped in menopause, some of your impetus for giving so much of your time and energy to others may also have faded. You didn't mention your body type, but if you happen to be an hourglass-shaped woman (or you were at one time) with big hips and full breasts, you may have had a high estrogen level when you were young, and now the loss of estrogen may be hitting you harder.

So many women juggle so much, just as you do. As part of the sandwich generation, we are squeezed between taking care of aging parents and mourning adult kids leaving home (or dealing with them boomeranging back); between needy partners and our own illnesses (as we live longer, we often live with something chronic, or our partners do); between economic challenges and changes at home or at work.

How about using this golden estrogen-dropping moment to put *yourself* on the top of your to-do list? This may feel different and difficult at first, but you deserve it, especially after your lifetime of giving and nurturing others. Not only that, if you don't stay focused on meeting your own needs more, you may risk illness, lack of stamina, growing dissatisfaction with your life, maybe even depression yourself. What good will you be then to your aging father or depressed husband?

This really can be your time to shine in new ways. At first, you may have to pretend you are taking care of someone else in order to arrange for your own self-care, like perhaps joining a gym, spending a day with girlfriends, planning a weekly date night with your husband (might do him a world of good, too), volunteering somewhere you enjoy, taking a class, learning a musical instrument or a new language, joining a cause you believe in, walking in nature—your options are limited only by your imagination.

And while you are thinking about it, perhaps give some thought to what

Dr. Dorree Says:

Women sometimes wear so many hats, they lose their heads! It helps to think of ourselves as well-rooted trees with branches that reach out to the world and up to the sky. If we aren't well-watered and well-nourished, our branches droop and our trunk dies. When we are well-fed, our branches can grow and we can reach for the sun. Nature can teach us so much about ourselves and life.

might be an appropriate next step for your dad. If it's not time for a nursing home, maybe adult day care would give him some more stimulation among people his age, while setting you free for a big chunk of the day. (Who knows, your father might even rekindle a bit of his own sex drive again, which would be a great pick-me-up for him.)

Let your heart guide you where you want to go and do things that make you smile.

QUESTION: *Ever since my wife stopped menstruating two years ago, the arguing has gotten really bad and I'm sick of it. I love my wife and I don't want to get divorced, I just want to stop fighting! I say it's because she's in menopause; she says it's because I'm a jerk. Who's right?*

— David, 54

Maybe you're both a little right. Actually, you sound like a caring guy in a lousy situation that you don't yet know what to do about. A menopausal woman isn't always a pure joy to live with. Couples often fight over the opening and closing of windows and the setting of the thermostat, or other such trivial annoyances, but when a woman is in menopause these fights can get really heated. She's too hot, she's too cold, and frankly, she's too much of a pain in the ass! Relationship problems can start or intensify during and after menopause, and your love connection can get strained. You didn't mention sex, but it wouldn't surprise us if that has taken a hike, too.

Chapters 5 and 6 are full of good ideas for how to communicate with each other better, build your bond, and have better sex. You might also consider short-term therapy to learn ways to work through this period. If your wife won't go with you, just go by yourself. She may follow in time, and in any case, you will probably find it useful.

Who's Sexy Now?

A friend recently said, "I don't feel sexy because I am not sexy. No amount of positive thinking is going to turn me into Madonna, not even on the inside."

If you don't feel your own sexy vibe anymore, there's probably more to the story than just biochemistry. It can be hard to feel your own sexiness when just about everywhere you go, society is telling you, either directly or indirectly, that you are too old, too ugly, too undesirable, or too over the hill. Until our culture starts valuing aging and respecting the sexuality of older women, wise women over 50 can benefit from being aware of what's happening and actively counterbalancing these negative ideas with positive self-messages and role models. Women at every age can and do masturbate regularly, have sexual fantasies, and enjoy sex. At every age, your body, though changed, is still sensual, interesting, sexy, and a great playground to explore.

In other words, you're still hot!

Women on Sex After 50

Gail Sheehy asked Gloria Steinem (whom Sheehy described as "not only the inspiration of the feminist movement" but also as "one of the most sexually animated women of her time") what sex was now like for her after 50. Steinem said: "Going to bed for two entire days and sending out for Chinese food was such an important part of my life, and it just isn't anymore. It's still there, but it's less important. I don't know how much of it is hormonal and how much is outgrowing it."

Or as Cora says: "The part about sending out for Chinese food still holds true, but with three teenagers still at home, I can barely remember the rest."

For Maria, desire has intensified: "Passion about my lover, if anything, is more intense than ever; it's the frequency that has not been sustained."

Tina: "With my kids gone, I feel more relaxed and more easily 'turned on.' Unfortunately, my husband seems less interested and that frustrates me and leaves me feeling lonely and discouraged."

Linda: "I love men, always have, always will. I prefer intercourse to masturbation every time."

Siegfried: "I don't have much sexual desire anymore and I find that relieving. My energies go elsewhere. I always wanted to sculpt, throw the wheel, or, to be more precise, be a potter. Now, instead of sex and spending so much time making others happy, all my energy and focus is spent with my arms up to my elbows in clay. I am at creative and spiritual peace."

Denise: "I think sex gets better with age. In the past

five years, I have done as I pleased when it came to sex. I have no one to answer to. I have all the fabulous affairs I could wish for and that feels liberating. I live every day to the fullest and I finally love my life"

Toni: "I am just as horny at sixty as I was at sixteen, but my guy considers me too old to be sexy!"

Jenny: "I am 78 and live alone. Male companionship is a bloody bore. I don't miss sex in any form and I will never marry again."

Roll Like a Role Model

Rather than comparing yourself to younger women (or yourself at a younger age), how about looking for strong, beautiful, and vibrant females over 50 to admire and perhaps even emulate? Perhaps you could visit women who are older and learn who they have become. Or you can look in books, magazines, movies, the arts, or public life. Your after-50 female can also be a fictional character or a real person. Some candidates to consider include:

- *Entertainers:* Meryl Streep; Joanne Woodward; Catherine Deneuve; Dame Helen Mirren; Dame Judith Dench; Dame Angela Lansbury; Diahann Carroll; Chita Rivera; Eartha Kitt; Ruby Dee; Oprah, Martha Graham; Sophia Loren; and Gina Lollobrigida.
- *Political Figures:* Ellen Johnson Sirleaf, Liberian president; Golda Meir, first president of Israel; Indira Gandhi, prime minister of India; Mary Robinson and Mary McAleese,

consecutive presidents of Ireland; Chandrika Kumaratunga, first female president of Sri Lanka; Corazon Aquino, first female president of the Philippines; Barbara Jordon, congressperson from Texas; Janet Reno, U.S. attorney general; Coretta Scott King; Jacqueline Kennedy Onassis; Empress Farah of Iran; Joan of Arc; and Aung San Suu Kyi, 1991 Nobel Peace Prize–winner.

- *Scientists and Mathematicians:* Marie Curie; Margaret Sanger; Bernadine Healy, physician and former head of the National Institutes of Health; Barbara McClintock, 1983 Nobel Laureate in Physiology/Medicine; and Dame Mary Lucy Cartwright, leading twentieth-century British mathematician.
- *Religious Leaders and Religious Educators:* Mother Teresa, Nobel Peace Prize–winner; Mary Baker Eddy, founder of the Christian Science movement; Rev. Katharine Jefferts Schori, first female bishop of the Episcopal Church; and Nischala Joy Devi, master teacher and international yoga advocate and pioneer.
- *Literary writers and characters:* Azar Nafisi, Iranian professor and author of *Reading Lolita in Tehran*; Isabel Allende, Chilean-American author, and one of her main literary characters, Inés Suárez; Mary Anne Evans, better known under the pen name George Eliot; Simone de Beauvoir, author of *The Second Sex*; Jane Austen and her characters; Toni Morrison, Nobel prize–winner and author; and Joyce Carol Oates, prolific author of over fifty novels and still producing.
- *Musicians:* Joni Mitchell; Joan Baez; Dame Kiri Te Kanawa, New Zealand opera singer; Madonna; "Mama"

Cass Elliot; Tina Turner; Cher; Patti LaBelle; Grace Slick; Billie Holiday; Jacqueline du Pré, cellist; Marin Alsop, first female conductor of the Baltimore Symphony Orchestra; and Clara Schumann, pianist.

- *Fashion:* Diane Von Furstenburg; Donna Karan; Eileen Fisher; and Betsey Johnson.
- *Entrepreneurs:* Oprah, Martha Stuart, Sheila Johnson, Meg Whitman, Carly Fiorina, Sallie Krawcheck

"A Woman of a Certain Age"

This in-vogue term was originally used to describe an unmarried woman or spinster. It later came to mean an older woman—although what exactly qualifies you to be officially "older" is not clear. So why use it at all? We don't say a "child of a certain age" or a "teenager of a certain age." If we take the pro-aging position, no woman is of a certain age. We are each precisely who we are at 50, 60, 70, 80, and beyond—without shame. Given that people over 50 now account for about a quarter of the U.S. population, how about we become leaders and explorers, instead of apologists? One's age can be anonymous, shameful, or a point of pride. After all, you made it this far and you're still rockin'.

Attitude Is Everything

Sex (alone or with a partner) is good for you—physically, mentally, and emotionally. If sex has become no fun or nonexistent, it will probably take some effort to get it back. If you don't make this effort, which of course is your choice, you will

Dr. Dorree Says:

It can be useful to pick a role model and really study her. What does (or did) she do to stay active and vital? How does she dress and carry herself. What are her interests and goals? These are people with problems and solutions, just like you and me, yet they achieve.

likely lose your sexuality entirely and maybe look like your great-great-grandmother before your time, which may be perfectly okay with you. Just be aware that whatever you do (or don't do), you are making a choice.

As with most things in life, attitude is everything. A good attitude on its own is not all you need, but without it, positive change is very difficult. If you don't have a good attitude about sex, where can you get one? How can you build your sexual self-esteem?

There are many entrance points to this ongoing process. For example, you could start by building your physical body and overall strength with great food and gradually increasing exercise. Or, if you are single, you could start by dating (see Chapter 7) and build your self-esteem when you discover that other people can be attracted to you, and you to them. Or you could start by learning to communicate more effectively with your partner (see Chapter 6) about what you want and need. Or you could simply begin by spending a little time alone and explaining to yourself that you are (simply by virtue of being alive) someone who deserves to be treated well by other people, including yourself. You may not like some parts of yourself or your body. So what? Nobody's perfect. What do you like about yourself? Start there.

Masturbation: The Gift You Give Yourself

QUESTION: *I don't see how this stuff about sex after 50 applies to me. I live alone. I don't date anyone, and I wouldn't know where to find someone if I wanted to. Am I really missing out?*

— GUILIA, 68

There are no sex rules for how you must live your life. On the other hand, just because it is okay doesn't necessarily mean it's good enough for you. Do you have any desire for desire? Would you like to find out?

Anyone who has never had an orgasm—as well as everyone who has—can benefit greatly from regular sexual activity on one's own. Masturbating regularly, even if you have a partner, is vital for keeping your sexual juices flowing. It brings blood and oxygen to your vagina and pelvic region, tones your internal muscles, and reminds your body that you are still fully alive from stem to stern.

Beyond the physical advantages, regular masturbation has many other great benefits as well. For one thing, it teaches you what you like and don't like sexually, and trains you to get very good at it. If you do find a partner (see Chapter 7 for ideas), you can share what you've discovered to help him or her learn how to give you deep satisfaction. Plus, touching yourself in ways that bring you pleasure is a way of being loving to yourself instead of just taking your body for granted. And most of all, lots of masturbation will help wake up the sexy part of you

Dr. Dorree Says:

Experiencing and enjoying sex is part of being fully alive. Do you really want to let it go, perhaps forever? If you do, that's fine. But if you don't want to let it go, you don't have to.

that may have dozed off recently—or perhaps a long time ago. Even for women whose sexuality is already wide awake, regular masturbation can keep you warmed up and ready to go.

Many women first learn about masturbation in tubs and showers. European women have the convenient bidets to help stimulate them. Jacuzzis and hot tubs with jets can also work wonders. Whatever the source, a steady flow of warm water, at an adjustable pressure, is a great way to get started. If you don't have a shower massager with a long, flexible hose, this might be a good time to get one. Set the water temperature as you like it (not too hot for delicate vaginal tissues) and experiment with different angles and settings. Stick with it until you have an orgasm (or run out of water!). If you don't have one the first time, that's fine. Keep it up and you might be surprised how your body will learn.

Your hand, or course, is always available. And a vibrator (see Chapter 9) can become your best electronic friend. Keep it plugged in bedside (perhaps tastefully hidden), so you can use it early and often, or late and often, as you wish. Unlike a shower, a plug-in vibrator can go as long as you like.

Too shy to masturbate, even alone? Are you aware that most people do it? It's true that self-pleasuring is practiced more by men than women (some guys enjoy it so freely they make it a hobby). But most women do masturbate, including up to 25 percent of women over the age of 70, according to early research. Many older women who do not have a partner or who have partners with illnesses or sexual dysfunctions, use masturbation as a replacement for intercourse. And mutual masturbation is a common sexual practice for many couples, with or without vaginal penetration.

So before you give up on ever having an orgasm, experiment

with a little quality time in the tub or with a vibrator. You can use bed or bath pillows to make yourself comfortable. Perhaps light a candle or two. Lock the door for added security and relax and enjoy yourself. Even if you don't hit that illusive Big O, don't pressure yourself; it will still feel really good!

Up Close and Personal:
Your Secret Anatomy of Sexual Pleasure

There is a lot more to a woman's sexual anatomy than meets the eye. In fact, most of the external and internal tissues that become aroused during sexual stimulation and make sex so pleasurable for a woman cannot be seen at all. Unlike for a man, whose singular sex organ is in full view and easily accessible, a woman's multiple sex parts are mostly hidden and largely unknown—even to most women.

If you aren't fully aware of what your exquisite external sex organs look like, you might find it fascinating to get a mirror and take a look. You will notice that your vagina has two sets of lips (labia), one smaller set inside another larger set, like flower petals. Near the top of the inner lips, above your urethral opening (where the pee comes out), is the hooded head of the clitoris.

What you cannot see, however, is all the rest of your sexually responsive and oh-so important sex parts. For example, although the head of the clitoris appears small, the full clitoris is actually much larger and more complex. In addition to the sensitive external head, there is also an internal clitoral shaft and two long clitoral "legs" that bracket the sides of the vaginal opening, along the pubic bone.

Sheri Winston, in her book called *Women's Anatomy of*

Arousal, describes and diagrams for us a wonderland of female erectile tissues and arousal network that few people have any idea exists, no less know how to fully stimulate and enjoy. Among the many sexually responsive structures hidden inside a woman's pelvis is the famous—and often misunderstood— G-spot. According to Winston and others and contrary to what most of us have been taught, the G-spot isn't really a specific "spot" at all. Rather than being a small bull's eye that must be precisely hit, Winston calls it a "groove tube," a spongy network of erectile tissue that lies between the urethra and the front wall of the vaginal canal. Without arousal, it's hard to feel. With arousal, there's no doubt about its succulence. Forget the debate about whether or not it exists. Play with it yourself or teach your partner how to play you well.

Some recent research indicates that a collagen injection, given under local anesthetic, in the area of the G-spot may enhance women's sexual pleasure. We don't know too many women who have done this procedure, which takes about 90 minutes and costs thousands of dollars. Follow-up studies are small, and it doesn't appear to work if sexual desire isn't also present. However, we predict more marvelous help for increased arousal will continue to be invented. Whatever it may be, we recommend that you are not the guinea pig and that you wait until the newly touted mysterious magic becomes a scientifically proven safe product.

Do keep in mind that not everyone's G-spot is a turn-on for them, which is why it helps to masturbate often so you can learn more about what you like—and keep your sex organs lively!

READER/CUSTOMER CARE SURVEY

We care about your opinions! Please take a moment to fill out our online Reader Survey at **http://survey.hcibooks.com**.

As a **"THANK YOU"** you will receive a **VALUABLE INSTANT COUPON** towards future book purchases

as well as a **SPECIAL GIFT** available only online! Or, you may mail this card back to us.

(PLEASE PRINT IN ALL CAPS)

First Name _____ MI. _____ Last Name _____

Address _____ City _____

State _____ Zip _____ Email _____

1. Gender
❑ Female ❑ Male

2. Age
❑ 8 or younger
❑ 9-12 ❑ 13-16
❑ 17-20 ❑ 21-30
❑ 31+

3. Did you receive this book as a gift?
❑ Yes ❑ No

4. Annual Household Income
❑ under $25,000
❑ $25,000 - $34,999
❑ $35,000 - $49,999
❑ $50,000 - $74,999
❑ over $75,000

5. What are the ages of the children living in your house?
❑ 0 - 14 ❑ 15+

6. Marital Status
❑ Single
❑ Married
❑ Divorced
❑ Widowed

7. How did you find out about the book?
(please choose one)
❑ Recommendation
❑ Store Display
❑ Online
❑ Catalog/Mailing
❑ Interview/Review

8. Where do you usually buy books?
(please choose one)
❑ Bookstore
❑ Online
❑ Book Club/Mail Order
❑ Price Club (Sam's Club, Costco's, etc.)
❑ Retail Store (Target, Wal-Mart, etc.)

9. What subject do you enjoy reading about the most?
(please choose one)
❑ Parenting/Family
❑ Relationships
❑ Recovery/Addictions
❑ Health/Nutrition
❑ Christianity
❑ Spirituality/Inspiration
❑ Business Self-help
❑ Women's Issues
❑ Sports

10. What attracts you most to a book?
(please choose one)
❑ Title
❑ Cover Design
❑ Author
❑ Content

TAPE IN MIDDLE; DO NOT STAPLE

BUSINESS REPLY MAIL
FIRST-CLASS MAIL PERMIT NO 45 DEERFIELD BEACH, FL

POSTAGE WILL BE PAID BY ADDRESSEE

Health Communications, Inc.
3201 SW 15th Street
Deerfield Beach FL 33442-9875

FOLD HERE

Comments

A Little Vaginal TLC

QUESTION: *I stopped menstruating two years ago and now I have no interest in sex. I use to enjoy making love. Now my vagina is dry and unresponsive. Will this ever change?*

—Kim, 54

Of course, it will change. *How* it will change is up to you. If you do nothing, it may progress in a direction you aren't wild about. Luckily, there are options.

Four out of five women report experiencing some sex problems during menopause, including vaginal dryness and unresponsiveness. For many, it's just a temporary downturn. For others, however, interest in sex completely dries up—literally. Here are some ways to care for your vagina.

Vaginal suppositories. Medications, such as prescription Vagifem or other localized estrogen boosters that don't go through the liver, can be effective for reversing a dry vagina. Many physicians believe that treating the issue closer to the source is less invasive and therefore better.

Kegel exercises. These are internal isotonic exercises that build strength in your pelvic floor muscles to support your organs and make orgasms more intense. Kegels are performed by repeatedly squeezing and releasing your innermost pelvic muscles as if you are trying to stop the flow of urine in mid-pee. Many women learn how to do this in preparation for childbirth. Pilates teaches this easily (and usually no one even knows it helps sex, often not even the instructor). The great thing about Kegels is you need no special equipment and you can do it anywhere—like while you're waiting in line to pick up a latte or your dry cleaning.

Pelvic floor therapy. This is a type of specialized physical therapy specifically for a vagina that has atrophied (become smaller) due to menopause or lack of sexual activity, or a vagina that is recovering from surgery, abuse, or other trauma. This physical therapy involves the repeated gentle stretching of the inside of the vagina—either with fingers or a dildo—so it can regain elasticity and size. People use physical therapy for all sorts of things, from back pain to recovering from knee surgery, so why not use it for pelvic rehab as well? This relatively recent treatment has proved highly successful for many women who are willing to do their homework and stick with the program.

Vagina Revival

Rhoda's marriage was dying. The relationship was beyond repair and she hadn't had sex, or even any desire for sex, for more than a year. Her vagina was dry and "asleep." Rhoda naturally assumed this was the end of the road, not only for her marriage, but for her sexuality. Six months after leaving her husband, Rhoda met a great guy and fell in love. She held off becoming sexually intimate with her new beau as long as she could. She dreaded having to confess to him that with her dry vagina she no longer enjoyed sex. When the time finally came, Rhoda was shocked to discover that her vagina was wide awake, plenty wet, and ready to go. They had passionate sex for many hours that night and after that, she was never dry again.

Dr. Dorree Says:

A woman can fake an orgasm, but she can't fake desire. If it's not there, her vagina is not going to open up, get wet, or perform on command. If it is there, there's little that stops a woman's passion.

Pills and Other Possibilities

Men have erectile dysfunction (ED) pills, women don't have a good one yet. How come? Well, we could say it's mostly because men conduct medical research and they are ignoring women, but that's not really true. In fact, scientists have been trying for years to come up with a way to help women come and new versions of a "pink Viagra" for women are being tested and are starting to be available. Soon, one of these pills will be shown to work better than another. We look forward to a great one coming along. But, as with all male libido enhancers, no doubt, desire will remain key. And as with all medications, there will be no perfect panacea, no one size fits all. No one pill that will work without interfering with some other prescription. Until the pink one comes along, some women have been known to try the already on the market blue male enhancement pills. (Whatever the color; if it works, great. Just use the same care as you would with any other medication.)

But beyond the pill quest is a bigger issue that no drug will even be able to address. For everyone, and for women especially, sex and desire are intertwined, and no one has figured out how to put emotional desire into a pill. Writers, such as Clarissa Pinkola Estes (*Women Who Run with the Wolves*) and many others, focus on sexuality and desire as it is integrated with a woman's body, heart, mind, and soul. Women often long for something more than what modern family life provides. Some modern women may secretly or unconsciously crave the freedom to return to the archetypical wild woman who gets to do what she

Dr. Dorree Says:

However you chose to do it, stoking the flames of your authentic desires also helps to turn up the heat in the bedroom, too.

wants when the spirit moves her and enjoys life more fully.

After 50, this may be your time to get reacquainted with that "wild" part of yourself. Many women do—and some choose to give up men or choose to relate to them differently. However, men, too, have longings and vulnerabilities that they don't express. How fortunate if both you and your changing man can take this second half of life's journey together. You may not have to travel very far afield. Your local house of worship, yoga or meditation center, university lecture series, or nature walks may all offer starting places for this kind of exploration. And, of course, good therapy may also help.

Seven Myths About Women After 50

Myth #1: Older women are lousy lovers. (**False.** For centuries, in many countries, it was expected that a young man would be initiated into the world of sexual pleasures by an older woman.)

Myth #2: Older women don't want sex as much as older men do. (**False.** Women just want more talk along with sex.)

Myth #3: Older women's sex drive diminishes more quickly than older men's. (**False.** It's just more complex.)

Myth #4: Older women don't want oral sex. (**False.** Some do, some don't.)

Myth #5: Older women don't fantasize. (**False.** Many have active fantasy lives.)

Myth #6: Older women must have romance to have sex. (**False,** though many do desire connection).

Myth #7: Older women lose their vaginal sensitivity. (**False.** It depends on the woman.)

Outer Beauty After 50

After menopause, many women gain weight, especially around the waist and hips, while thinner women may become somewhat bonier, losing fat and collagen from their breasts and face. As the great French actress and classic beauty Catherine Deneuve is alleged to have said, "As women age they either have to give up on their face or their derriere; it's hard to keep both." Either way, enjoy what you have. Here are some issues to consider.

Hair challenges. Hair, and what to do with it, is usually at the top of the list of after-50 beauty woes. We often become very attached to our hair and may even feel that our identity is linked to it, so when it goes grayer, gets thinner, or changes texture, it can be hard to wrap your head around it. If you have long hair, should you cut it? Will it really look better shorter, or do you think you are just "too old" for long locks? Why should it matter? We say just wear your hair (if you have enough left) any way you wish! Wigs are an option, too, if you feel so inclined. Diet changes work for some and a few women have gone the hair plug route. It's your head. Do with it as you wish.

Skin care. Skin care is also a concern for many women, especially as they age, and accounts for a big part of the multi-billion-dollar cosmetic industry. But the expensive stuff is often no better than less costly options. The key is to hydrate. Use makeup any way you wish, but remember more is not always best. Steer clear of your daughter's makeup (and your mom's). You can skip makeup altogether or consider a makeup-makeover. Most good department stores have cosmetic departments that offer makeovers free by appointment in the hope that you will buy some of their products (you don't have to).

Nonsurgical procedures and products. Treatments to tighten the face and minimize wrinkles include Botox and wrinkle or line fillers, facials, peels, dermabrasion, laser treatments, and other face work that can give you significant, but temporary, changes. Be wary of treatments offered by hair salons and unlicensed people. This is your face! And your money. Get someone who knows what they are doing. Acupuncture can also be effective for relaxing lines and smoothing the face. And you can buy exfoliating products and gizmos that remove the top layer of dead skin cells, which you can use in the privacy of your own home. We prefer green or environmentally sound cosmetic products that don't add more junk to your system or the planet. There are several websites (see the Resources section at the back of the book) that rate products that are considered better for you and save the earth as well.

Surgical procedures. Cosmetic surgery has changed dramatically in recent years, offering many more options that are less extensive and less costly than in the past. Nose reshaping, removal of fat by liposuction, and breast enlargements and reductions are among the most popular procedures. If you are very large breasted, minimizing the weight in front can decrease the strain on your back (especially if you are already dealing with osteoporosis or spinal compression). If you are looking to enlarge your breasts, keep in mind that many men who love them say that fake boobs just don't feel the same as the real thing. Facial cosmetic surgery is also an option. But remember, all surgery is serious, especially if you have general anesthesia. Sometimes poor results can happen to good people. Sometimes the aesthetics look good but don't feel good, especially to your partner.

Going au naturel. Going the natural route is just fine, too. Hold your head up proudly and love your body. Self-esteem and confidence ultimately grow and glow from the inside out. Take care of your spirit, your mind, and your body. Build and enjoy a community of friends and family, challenge your mind with new adventures, and nurture yourself like you would a newborn baby. Nothing beats eating well, staying hydrated, and being physically active to bring out the beauty in any women at any age.

To Coif or Not to Coif?

Young, hip women aspiring to pubescence tend to shave or wax their pubic hair, or even go permanently bare. Women around 50 know this is common, especially for those under 50, but don't know what to do—to remove or not to remove? They tend to straddle the issue—some trim it, some remove it entirely, and some let it grow naturally. Women over 60 usually don't even think about it unless their daughters talk very openly or they travel in unusual circles. They may try it, but feel strangely naked without their protective bush, and besides when it grows back it itches. Older women may wonder if the guy drops out, is it because I didn't bare all. Whatever you choose, unless you are a rare nudist, few in our society find stragglers along a bathing suit crotch line a turn-on.

Inner Beauty After 50

Whatever beauty work you do on the outside, remember that our bodies are like used cars whose parts do wear down over time. Inner beauty, on the other hand, can grow in your wonderful "bonus years." If you've lived your life consciously all along, great. If not, you have more opportunities now than ever before to come home to yourself and be more comfortable in your own skin. Much of it has to do with keeping your mind open to new people, ideas, and attitudes. It can be as simple as holding your head high, putting your best foot first, and looking forward eagerly to everything each day has to offer.

Once you begin to find the inner peace that comes from self-acceptance and joyful living, it can light you up from the inside more than any fancy skin product or face-lift, and it can be yours forever. Sometimes therapy can help you get there, as can eating well, living well, being physically active, spending time with people who enjoy life, and of course, keeping sex alive.

FOUR

MALE MEN-O-MORPH AND SEX FOREVER
Performance Power Customized

Okay guys, this one's for you.

We know you like to cut to the chase, so here it is: Sex for most men after 50 is different from the hormone-driven sex of your youth. Not necessarily worse or better, but like most things in life, surely different. So what are you going to do about it? Viagra and other erectile dysfunction (ED) pills don't always work and no one is getting any younger. If you don't want to give up sex, the only real solution to dealing with change is more change: a new way of being sexual that is still damn good, just different.

You and Your "Best Friend"

Years ago, it used to be so simple. When you first found your penis it likely became a major preoccupation, perhaps even your best buddy. Perhaps you masturbated with a *Playboy* magazine hidden under your bed. Once pimples appeared, so did the girls (or guys), and sex went from a solo act to a team sport, ushering in all the joys and complexities that sexual relationships bring. As an adult, married or single, gay or straight, you found your way and may have enjoyed years of reliable sexual activity. Your powerful penis could be counted on for pretty much delivering on cue.

But then, starting around 50, your trustworthy friend may have stopped performing as reliably as before. The Viagra, Cialis, and Levitra ads tell you this is common—but it's not common for you. Maybe you feel confused and alone. Maybe you wonder if you are over the hill and just too old for sex. Maybe your performance anxiety is so high you simply worry about trying again.

Actually, sexuality never dies. Men can be sexual at every age and stage of life, although sex usually changes significantly after 50. Compared to women, you are at a disadvantage in seeing this coming. Women have the experience of menopause to clearly announce their big sex transformation. Bells go off, or at least hot flashes begin; blankets get tossed off; they dress in layers like their teenage daughters; tempers grow short; and emotions run high. Any man who has lived with a menopausal woman knows that her "big change" is no walk in the park.

Your man-changes, however, are more gradual. They just sort of sneak up slowly on you. You may hardly notice them at first, or maybe you just chalk it up to stress at work or problems at home. After a while, your changing penis performance may become a more noticeable issue, perhaps even a daily worry. It may seem like your reliable buddy is letting you down. Maybe it won't get quite as hard or get hard as often as it once did, and if it does, it may not stay hard as long as you wish. But the great men-o-morph that men experience in their 50s, 60s, and beyond needn't be the beginning of the end of your sex life. Believe it or not, sex now can be even better than before—once you understand that your body and life are changing and you discover how to ride it for all it's worth.

So let's bypass the super media hype about Viagra and skip the phony penis enlargement pills, and get real about what is actually going on and how you can start using it to your advantage. Even if you've been having sex all your life, there is still more to learn. Information is power, and at each new age, you are getting more powerful than ever before. Consider this equivalent to graduate school classes in sex that you didn't even know you wanted to take.

What's Happening to My Penis?

QUESTION: *I've noticed lately that my penis seems a bit smaller (or maybe just my belly is bigger?) and it doesn't get as hard as it used to, which is embarrassing in bed. Do I have erectile dysfunction?*

—DAVE, 56

What's happening to your penis is what's happening to all of you: your body and your life are changing. This is normal and natural. One reason for the change is that your body's production of the male sex hormone testosterone is gradually declining. Testosterone begins to fall in the late 30s and early 40s, and diminishes at a constant rate thereafter, in the range of about 1.6 percent per year, according to longitudinal data from the 2002 Massachusetts Male Aging Study. As testosterone declines, estrogen creeps up, causing fat deposits and even breast development.

Normally declining testosterone may actually be protective for men, perhaps even helping to extend life. But just as puberty took some time to get used to, so will this big change. Testosterone is what made you into a boy instead of a girl. It lowered your voice and put hair on your face and body as a teenager. And testosterone is what made the pursuit of sex a central focus of your adult life. So naturally, falling testosterone levels after 50 have a big impact on how you feel about yourself, as well as how you function. The physical effects of declining sex hormones can include slower metabolism, weight gain, less drive to be competitive, easier fatigue, erections that seem smaller and less rock-hard than before and less forceful ejaculations.

Except in rare cases, gradually declining testosterone after age 50 is not a medical problem. What the media ads tout as "erectile dysfunction" or ED is actually quite normal for men over 50 and if viewed this way, does not necessarily require any medical treatment (although you may choose to use a little help from a prescription buddy or other sex aid on occasion— or often).

For a man over 50 whose penis won't do what he wants it to do, all this natural change might feel like a real bummer. But there's a silver lining to getting older: Instead of judging yourself in comparison to your youth, you can allow your attitude to shift. Your seemingly wayward penis is actually giving you a wonderful chance to experience even better sex than before. (Really, we are not making this up!) But granted, it can take some getting used to.

Before we get to that later in this chapter, let's see how your changing penis measures up against the rest.

Penis Size: The Hard Facts

A website for a penis-enlargement patch promises you can "realize total and absolute power and domination in bed with your newfound penis size and sexual performance." One can almost imagine a mad scientist pulling open his white lab coat to pour a flask of magic miracle-grow on his own swelling member and shouting "Eureka!" as he dials the *Guinness Book of World Records.*

Since the beginning of time, men have equated penis size with masculinity and power. Just look at ancient art to validate what we are saying. Even today, our society is still quite penis-focused. As a kid, you may have lived in a time and place where the freedom of pissing contests and "circle jerks" was the norm. Your "peter meter" was exposed and judged. It's common for adolescent boys to measure and compare the heft of their maturing wands to see who has the biggest, and men of all ages wonder if their male members make the grade. Any adult male who has been in a locker room knows this to be so.

In truth, penises come in a normal range of lengths, and size does not make much difference. So what nature endowed you with is just fine. While a few women do prefer bigger penises, either for the aesthetics or the fit, the vast majority of partners say size does not matter. As long as it fits inside a vagina, it does the job. Still, psychologically, size does matter to many men (and some women, as well). So what exactly constitutes a big penis? Let's whip out the facts:

- The average adult penis is five to six inches long, *erect.*
- A flaccid male organ averages about three and a half inches long.

- The quest for penis enlargement via all manner of bogus patches and pills is futile, despite ads that claim you can "drastically enlarge penis length and width to sizes previously thought impossible!" (Note that the last word is the only point of fact.)
- Penis pumps can help men with medical problems—such as complications after prostate cancer surgery—achieve erections, but they are not designed to super-size a normal male member.

How Long Can You Last?

After penis size, the next big concern for many men is how long they can go before coming. Medical researchers say premature ejaculation (PE) is the most common sexual complaint of younger men, affecting 25 to 40 percent of men of all ages in the U.S. But what exactly is it? Medically, premature ejaculation (also called rapid ejaculation, rapid climax, premature climax, or early ejaculation) has no precise definition.

Notable sex researchers William Masters and Virginia E. Johnson believed that a man suffers from premature ejaculation if he ejaculates before his sex partner achieves orgasm in more than half of their sexual encounters. But what if your partner takes an hour to come? Is that still PE? Others say a man has PE if he ejaculates within two minutes of penetration. But a survey by Alfred Kinsey in the 1950s demonstrated that three quarters of men ejaculate within two minutes of penetration in over half of their sexual encounters.

Self-reported surveys say up to 75 percent of men ejaculate within ten minutes of penetration. Today, most sex therapists define premature ejaculation as an orgasm that occurs when a lack of ejaculatory control interferes with sexual or emotional well-being in one or both partners. That's about as vague as it can be, but this is a time to applaud being vague because it's a positive message that says it's good if it works for you, as

Dr. Dorree Says:

Unless you make your living as a porn star, quality trumps quantity. How you use your penis is far more important than how big it is.

opposed to the more negative judgments that abound.

Because there is great variability in both how long it takes men to ejaculate and how long both partners want intercourse to last, researchers have been trying to form a more quantitative definition of premature ejaculation. Current evidence supports the idea that an "intravaginal ejaculation latency time" (meaning, the time from when you insert your penis into a vagina, or other orifice, to the time you have an orgasm) of less than about one and a half minutes may be considered premature ejaculation.

But like everything else involving sex, there's a lot more to the story than you can figure out with a ruler and a stopwatch. In fact, what the medical community calls a "problem" is really in the eye (or between the sheets) of the beholder. Some men who routinely ejaculate in less than a minute do not think they have a problem, while others may be able to last for twenty minutes or more and still say they have premature ejaculation. In truth, the time from erection to ejaculation can last anywhere from mere seconds to multiple minutes and still is perfectly normal. Whether or not it is a "problem" depends on a man's sexual satisfaction and his perception of his ability to control the timing of his ejaculation.

The Penis Pinch

If premature ejaculation is a concern for you, here's a technique you can try. During arousal and with an erection, either you or your partner can gently pinch the penis just above the scrotum. (It's physically easier and more fun if your partner is the one. See chapters 5 and 6 for more ideas.) By restricting the outflow of semen (ejaculation), this also slows the draining of blood from the chambers of the penis, which helps maintain an erection. As pressure and desire build, and when the time is right, release and enjoy!

Dr. Dorree Says:

Most premature ejaculation is due to anxiety. Sometimes it is physiological, but more often there is something in the bedroom that is making a man feel anxious or insecure. If a comprehensive physical exam rules out medical problems, maybe your relationship needs a tune-up. Decide which way to go (couples counseling or a new partner). A willing and trusted partner can do wonders to help your penis relax and prolong your pleasure.

Where Erections Come From

Most people tend to think sex begins and ends in the genitals when, in fact, sex starts in the brain. What we think about, including how we feel about ourselves, our partner, our fantasies, and—for men especially—what they see or think of visually, creates desire. In turn, the feeling of desire kicks off a series of physiological responses. In men, the head tells the heart to pump harder, getting the blood flowing to the penis. Vascular vessels inside the chambers of the penis begin to fill with blood and to expand. Presto, you've got an erection.

As you age, the connections between your head and your penis may not work as smoothly as when you were younger. Anxiety, anger, frustration, or just plain worrying about performance can get in the way. Illnesses, such as diabetes and high blood pressure, can impact your erections and ejaculations. And prescription medicines, such as antidepressants and many others, can interfere with sexual performance. (For details about how to have great sex despite illness, see Chapter 8.)

Even if all systems are go, it is perfectly normal and natural for a man over 50 to have erections that are not as rock-hard and do not last as long as before. That's because with added years, the blood chambers inside your penis do not fill with blood as completely, nor stay filled for as long as they used to. There is nothing wrong with you in the least; it's just the natural progression of life. The good news is with some new information and new thinking, like the ideas in this book, you can have still great sex at every age.

The Angle of the Dangle

Some men become concerned if their erect penis lists to the left or the right. A "bent nail" happens when the chambers of the penis fill unevenly with blood during arousal. But slanting to one side has no effect on how good your penis feels to your partner. Regardless of size, speed, or slant, the male member is perfectly designed to deliver lively sperm to a woman's receptive egg and continues to work the same way even if making babies is no longer part of the program. Most erect penises tilt about thirty degrees to the vertical, just the right angle to match the typical tilt of a woman's vagina. A well-aimed penis not only delivers sperm efficiently, it is also correctly poised to stimulate the clitoris and vagina during intercourse.

Older Men Often Get the Short End of the Stick

The number of men over 50 will exceed fifty million by the end of 2010, yet the health of older men has long been ignored by medical researchers, health clinicians, policymakers, and most unfortunately, the men themselves. Like women, men face many perplexing, normal body changes as they grow older, as well as an array of medical disorders linked to aging. It can be very confusing at times. Unlike women, men are far more likely to ignore their health, and many avoid the doctor's office like the plague, waiting for major health problems to seriously interfere with their daily lives before seeking help. Most guys are unaware of how many health problems and medications can potentially affect their sex lives.

Why not be proactive instead? As you get older and wiser, now is a good time to use all of the tools at your disposal so you can have great sex for the rest of your life. A good place to start is with a comprehensive physical to rule out or catch any hidden health challenges. Go once a year, perhaps around the time of your birthday as a special present to yourself and those you love. And seek medical advice as soon as something unusual comes up. Why wait for molehills to become mountains? But don't expect the doctor to handle it all for you. You may have to do some research about your particular health and sex challenges by reading books, visiting websites, and talking to other health professionals.

Many Prostate Problems Are Normal

The media is constantly telling men that their prostates are enlarged. But if you read the ads closely you can end up more confused than ever. After 50, many men often have prostate issues that, while rarely life threatening, can impact daily life. The prostate is a walnut-sized gland located just below the bladder. The two lobes of the prostate that surround the urethra help squeeze semen through the penis during sexual climax. For reasons no one definitively knows, it is very common for the prostate to enlarge as men age, a condition doctors call benign prostatic hyperplasia or hypertrophy (BPH). Although not a disease, BPH puts pressure on the bladder and can slow the flow of sperm through the penis. You may find yourself running off to the bathroom more often, even waking up in the middle of the night to pee. Prostate enlargement can also affect the hardness of your erections, as well as the speed and volume of your ejaculations.

While prostate enlargement is not in itself a medical disease, it can be associated with rare but serious health problems, such as some cancers. While most prostate cancer progresses so slowly that most men die with it, not from it, there are other more aggressive cancers that can shorten your life—which is why a good physical once a year is a smart way to go. Odds are very good that you just have garden-variety prostate enlargement and at some point it may start affecting your penis.

If BPH is a common and even natural part of life for older men, then expecting your penis to behave as if you don't have it is not being respectful to yourself. Prostate enlargement is just one of the things many guys naturally encounter during this phase of life, along with a tendency toward weight gain, less stamina, possibly some short term memory loss, and for some, a bit more anxiety, depression, and irritability—all of which can adversely affect sex. Feeling bad about yourself because of these

normal changes is neither fair nor productive. Better to understand what is happening to your changing body, and learn how
to continue to have terrific sex now.

Man Boobs Happen

QUESTION: *What's up with my chest? I'm embarrassed to say this,*
but I feel like I need a bra.

—LEONARD, 60

This is one of those big secrets that men rarely, if ever, talk
about, even men who may get together to chat weekly, play
cards together, talk about their business issues or illnesses, or
brag about conquests yet to be made. Actually, some men do
wear tight-fitting undershirts to minimize their breasts. Falling
testosterone after 50 tends to lower metabolism and increase
body fat. Because fat produces small amounts of estrogen and
because there's a bit less testosterone available to offset estrogen's effects, some men develop fuller breasts. A slight tip in a
man's estrogen-testosterone balance (toward estrogen) may also
partially explain why some men gravitate toward more affection as they age.

For women, the estrogen-testosterone balance tips slightly
more toward testosterone after 50, just enough to make some
women more assertive. Maybe that's why some say "time is the
great equalizer."

Eating well, staying active and especially exercising the
upper body musculature can help tame your man boobs and
keep you out of a bra (unless you like that sort of thing; then
by all means, enjoy!).

Midlife Crisis or Male Menopause?

QUESTION: *I've been feeling pretty lousy lately. I'm fat, tired all the time, and can't keep a hard-on to save my life. I'm bored at work, my marriage is in a rut, and it feels like life has passed me by. I know that men have less testosterone after age 50, but this seems like more than that. Am I having a midlife crisis or is it male menopause?*

—DARNEL, 57

There are no simple answers. As with women, the line between physiology and psychology blurs during a man's big midlife sex change. Just as puberty was a monumental transition, midlife is also very challenging for most people. Starting within five or ten years of age 50, men begin to notice both physical and psychological changes. Some people adapt to these changes reasonably well and accept them as part of aging. Others find them more difficult to deal with. Most are due to our naturally declining sex hormones that keep us from functioning as we did when we were younger. Other causes include decreased blood flow to the genitals, slower nerve function, and less elastic erectile tissue. There could be other reasons as well, such as diabetes and depression, which you may not know you have unless you get checked out by a doctor or other healthcare provider. (See Chapter 8 for more about sex and illness.)

Beyond physical causes, how you feel about yourself or your partner can also have an impact on how your penis performs. Some men who can achieve erection and ejaculation when they are by themselves can have a harder time when they are around a vagina. This can happen if a man is distrustful of women in general, if he is especially interested in one woman in particular and feels there is a lot riding on his performance, or if he is under significant stress at home or at work. Anything that prompts the body's adrenal glands to put out extra adrenaline can deflate a hard-on before orgasm. Among many other effects, this hormone opens up the valves in the penis's erection chambers, which causes the blood to flow out prematurely so the penis becomes flaccid.

Reducing stress in your life may do wonders for your health, happiness, and sex life. Instead of, or in addition to, buying an expensive sports car as a midlife crisis salve, you may want to consider investing in your relationship with a romantic getaway or short-term couples counseling, and investing in yourself by eating healthy foods in reasonable quantities and finding a moderate exercise that you can enjoy, like walking, swimming, biking, tennis, or whatever floats your boat (and makes your penis happy).

The real kick in the pants about stress is that a man's body can actually get into the habit of releasing adrenaline during sex, and this deflates your penis automatically, even when you are no longer stressed! In that case, you may want to try some relaxation techniques to retrain your mind and body.

Even some medications can cause trouble in bed. The *Journal of the American Medical Association* estimates that a shocking 25 percent of all sex performance problems in men are caused by the pills they consume. Take Marty, for example. For many months, Marty just couldn't stay hard when making love with his wife. He had no trouble getting an initial erection but soon his flag would be at half-mast. The couple was close to giving up on intercourse entirely when Marty's wife read an article about how some heart medicines can disrupt sex. Marty asked his doctor to try him on another medicine, and within a week, he was back in action in bed. At 59, Marty was never going to compete sexually with a younger version of himself, but by paying closer attention to the side effects of his medications, he was able to enjoy a new sexual beginning with his wife. To his surprise, she later told him she actually preferred his less forceful and slower love making because it helped her feel closer to him.

Why Not Just Pop a Pill?

QUESTION: *I am tired of feeling like a loser in bed. I am tempted to try one of those erectile dysfunction drugs. Should I?*

—BARRY, 65

Whether your penis is hard or soft, in or out, up or down, you are not a loser. You are more than your penis! If getting and maintaining an erection is worrying you, there are many approaches and aids you can try, including erectile dysfunction (ED) medications. But don't go into any treatment blind.

Watch a football game or other sports event on TV and the multiple ads make it all seem so easy. Just pop a pill and soon you'll be humping like you're 25 again. Or, better yet, take it every day so you'll always be "ready." Tons of money is poured into those ads in the hopes of making you believe that all you need is the right time, place, person—and the right pill—and presto, everything's great. In reality, it's not that simple. We want you happy and satisfied, not disappointed. These medications don't always work for everyone, or work equally well each time they are used.

Most ED drugs work by enhancing the effects of nitric oxide, a blood gas that relaxes penile blood vessels and allows blood to enter more freely, making an erection possible, but not creating one. For that you need desire and sexual stimulation—two things you cannot get in a pill. Drug side effects can include headache, flushing, nasal congestion, indigestion, urinary tract infections, diarrhea, backaches, vision problems, and even blindness (rare). Erectile dysfunction medicines can take up to an hour to take effect, cost $10 to $14 a pill, and don't always work. Many other things besides penile blood flood can impact your sexuality and performance, like how you feel about yourself and your partner. Even if you can get a harder penis after popping a pill, do you really want to try to Viagra your way out of a bad relationship? Can you?

Besides not always working, ED drugs can interfere with other medications, cause unwanted side effects, and may have unknown negative health impacts with long-term use. What good is it if you get a great hard-on now and next week your leg falls off? We joke; but seriously, who really knows what effects these drugs will have down the road?

Also keep in mind that no potency-enhancing drug can ever create the most fundamental requirement for any erection, which is *desire*. Maybe that explains why, according to some studies, 42 percent of men who try ED drugs stop using them. About half who quit say the treatments just didn't work. Could it be because Viagra, Cialis, and Levitra have no impact on emotions or relationships that may be affecting sexual functioning?

Erectile dysfunction drugs are huge moneymakers for pharmaceutical companies who spend millions trying to convince you that you desperately need them. They play on men's normal insecurities and push an unrealistic ideal of trying to maintain youthful momentum at every age, which is ridiculous.

We also have to question if this is a strictly Western cultural view of masculinity, where men are defined, at least in part, by the strength of their hard-ons. In many Eastern cultures, men enjoy sex at every stage of life without taking a single Western pharmaceutical. If anything, this new stage of gradually declining sex hormones after 50 is a golden opportunity—not to chase the past, but to embrace new wisdom and insight, and to enjoy sex, sensuality, and intimacy in new and exciting ways. Midlife is a time of reflection, redefinition, and even self-acceptance—not an illness to be fixed with a pill. The more a man worries about his erections, the less likely his penis will do what he wants it to do. Ultimately, he will come to accept his changing life and body, with or without the pills.

Of course, if you want to and it works for you, then try an ED drug. If one pill doesn't work, try another kind before you move on to investigate medical or relationship issues. When these pills work, they can make a world of difference. Some men (and their partners) swear by them.

Reggie beams when he talks about how after taking Cialis over a weekend vacation, both he and his live-in lover wound up in the same bathtub making mad passionate love. Isaiah kept his Viagra in the drawer next to his bed and the close proximity provided enough comfort and reassurance so that he never actually needed to take it. Orlando tried Viagra and hated the blue haze. He switched to Levitra and found new joy in bed.

Still, it's important to keep in mind that not being able to achieve and maintain the kind of erections you had when you were younger is usually not a medical problem; it's just a normal part of your ever-evolving life. The one thing sure to make a guy feel inadequate is to continually compare himself to the stud-muffin performance memories of his hormone-high youth. As one sexually active 72-year-old man said, "The toughest part isn't physical, but my memories and expectations. It's hard not getting hard!"

One of the best ways to deal with a penis that isn't doing exactly what you want it to do is to relax and accept yourself and your partner as you both are now. With or without an ED drug, consider taking the time to enjoy yourself and your partner without comparisons to others or to the past. And give up unrealistic demands for the future. Slip between your sheets with a be-here-now attitude and enjoy the marvelous sensations of being naked and alive. You never know what might pop up!

True Erectile Dysfunction

Even though most men who have less than rock-hard erections are perfectly normal and do not have a medical problem, there are some times when a man actually does have erectile dysfunction, which is defined as the inability to attain and maintain an erection sufficient for sexual intercourse at least 25 percent of the time. Either the penis doesn't get hard enough, or it gets hard but softens too soon. (The problem generally comes on gradually. Sudden erection difficulties are usually not true ED.)

True erectile dysfunction can be due to diabetes, kidney disease, atherosclerosis, prostate cancer, vascular disease, multiple sclerosis, alcoholism, nerve or blood vessel damage, scarring of penile tissue, smoking, obesity, abnormally low testosterone, and psychological issues. Even lack of sexual activity can cause ED. Months or years of no activity, with no regular blood flow to the penis, can make it difficult to jump-start your penis again.

Diagnostic assessments may include physical examination, blood tests, saliva tests, blood flow tests, and nocturnal tumescence tests (to see if you get an erection while sleeping). Treatments for ED range from oral drugs and penile injections to testosterone supplementation, sex therapy, surgery, and mechanical devices. When testosterone is abnormally low, supplemental testosterone in the form of a topical skin gel or daily intramuscular injection can help boost your libido and improve your ability to get and keep erections. Although no one knows precisely how testosterone alleviates ED, at least one study suggests that using testosterone gel along with the ED drug Viagra may be helpful for men with borderline low testosterone levels who don't respond to the drug alone.

Sometimes, when neither drugs nor hormones, alone or in combination, can effectively treat ED, some men turn to the . . .

Bionic Penis to the Rescue!

Men who can't or don't want to use medications and hormones can chose various mechanical devices to assist them in producing or maintaining an erection. A *penile band* (available without prescription under the name Actis and Erexel) can be fastened around the base of an erect penis to prevent blood from leaving the chambers of the penis too soon.

Or you can use a *vacuum erection device*. By inserting your non-erect penis into an airtight plastic cylinder and pumping the air out with a manual or battery-operated handheld pump, blood flows into the chambers of the penis, and like magic, you have a hard-on. Once achieved, you fit a rubber ring around the base of the penis (see pg. 103) and enjoy. The erection lasts until the ring is removed. Some men find the pump bothersome and have minor side effects, such as bruising and difficulty ejaculating. Still, it's a hard-on.

Two kinds of *surgical implants* are sometimes used when no other treatment succeeds. The first type consists of two pencil-thin silicone rods surgically implanted in the penile shaft, causing it to remain permanently erect (although it can be pointed down along the thigh to conceal it under clothing). The second type implants inflatable cylinders inside the penis that are attached to a tiny pump located in the scrotum. When the man wants an erection, he simply squeezes the pump, pushing saline fluid into the cylinders to create an erection. This generates a more natural feeling hard-on than silicone rods, but it is more prone to complications, such as infection or malfunction.

Are such treatments worth it? Some people think so. After prostate surgery, Phil made the difficult decision to undergo a second surgery to get an implant. During the months of his healing process, he continually questioned the wisdom of his choice. Then one morning he had intercourse with his wife, and although ejaculation is not an option, he lasted as long as he wished. After fifteen minutes, all his doubts disappeared. Phil and his wife were both very happy.

How Do I Know?

QUESTION: *Lately I can't get it up like I used to. How do I know if I have a normal, over-50 penis that just isn't going to get as hard as it used to, or if I have true erectile dysfunction?*

—RICKY, 54

As with so many things in life after 50, there are no easy answers. A medical checkup can be a good place to start. If you already know you have a medical problem or you take prescription medications of any kind, ask your doctor if your illness or treatment can affect sexual performance. You might be surprised by what you learn. Chapters 5 and 8 may help you with new ways to enjoy sex no matter what your penis is doing.

On the other hand, if you take no medications and have no known illnesses, you can reasonably assume that you don't have ED and your penis is just doing it's natural over-50 thing. Why fight it when you can enjoy it?

Penis Power: Less Performance, More Pleasure

Despite sometimes being referred to as a "nail" or a "bone" or some other tough terminology, the truth is that a man's penis is a highly delicate part of his being that responds with great sensitivity to both touch and emotion. Erections come and go, during sex and during sleep. Men can have many sexual sensations that go beyond their transient erections, yet they generally do not explore these with their partners. Instead, most men tend to follow the prescriptive foreplay-penetration-orgasm pattern learned in their youth, touted in the media, and seen in pornography.

All of this is very "erection focused" and can make any man worry about getting it up, keeping it up, and performing sexually. Though many men love "pussy," for psychological and cultural reasons a woman's vagina can be an intimidating place for some. Add to that the fact that many women expect their partners to take full responsibility for bringing them to orgasm. The pressures on a man in bed can be enormous. Just the process of putting on a condom, even with a partner's help, can create anxiety for some men and lead to the loss of erection. And anything that makes a man think he can't perform, often becomes true. That's why the semisoft erections men often have after 50 can be so vexing. The equipment seems to be "broken." But is it really?

John, a 57-year-old construction manager, says he used to think so, but now he's beginning to change his mind. "Psychologically, it was a real downer when I first started noticing my erection problems about eight years ago, and it stayed a real downer for a long time. But when I started focusing only on the physical sensations, I had to admit that having an erection that is not as hard as it used to be actually feels— can I even say this?—it actually feels a little *better* than when I was younger. I never thought I'd ever say this, but it feels really good when it's not completely hard, especially during oral sex. I didn't expect that!"

Erection and vaginal penetration are only a small part of the wide spectrum of sexual pleasures that a man can experience. Take anal stimulation, for example. Research shows that many men have an often unspoken desire to be touched and even penetrated anally (possibly by a finger or sex toy). Just inside the anus in men is an area near the prostate that if stimulated can lead to intense pleasure and even orgasm. In fact, most men enjoy having their testicles, perineum, and their entire genital area stimulated.

In truth, all of a man's body can be an erogenous zone. The skin is the largest sex organ and is often neglected. Shifting your focus from penetration and performance to relaxation and pleasure can make sex a whole lot more enjoyable, with or without an orgasm.

Master of Masturbation

QUESTION: *My wife doesn't understand why I still masturbate almost every day, even though we have sex pretty regularly. I think it makes her jealous, although she denies it. How can I make her understand it is not a rejection of her? I just like masturbating.*

—JUAN, 66

Most men have two separate sex lives, one with a partner and one alone. Men enjoy masturbating because they can fantasize about whatever they want and there is no pressure to perform. Masturbation is good for men (and women) and keeps us sexually healthy, both physically and mentally. You know exactly what you like. Plus, it can often be quick and easy. No foreplay or conversation necessary. Most men continue to masturbate, even when they have regular sex with a partner.

Some men are more relaxed when they masturbate and may not be willing or able to be as relaxed and open with their partners. Sex for one may feel less intimidating or may be a way to avoid being vulnerable with another person. For maximum sexual pleasure, it is great to have both—good sex alone and good sex together. No need to give up jerking off. At the same time, perhaps adding more intimacy with your partner would help you both feel closer and result in better sex.

One option is to include your wife or partner some (not necessarily all) of the time when you masturbate. Some women and men find it a great turn-on to watch a man pleasure himself. Or you could experiment with both of you masturbating together, side by side or at least in the same room. In some ways, masturbating in the presence of another person can be more intimate than intercourse because it can be less of a performance and perhaps an opportunity for a different type of closeness.

Or you can simply continue to masturbate on your own when your partner is not around. If it bothers her or him, be discreet.

Your Big Head Is More Powerful than Your Little Head

QUESTION: *My wife and I have been happily married for forty years. I still think she is beautiful and find her very sexy, but the pizzazz is gone from the bedroom for both of us. I can't keep an erection as well as I used to and sex is starting to feel more like work than fun. What can we do?*

—DERRICK, 68

This could be an excellent time to learn some new things about yourself and sex that you might not have known before. For starters, contrary to all our Madison Avenue and media myths that part of you probably believes, the performance of your penis does not determine who you are or how good sex feels. What you think and feel is what matters most to your sexuality, not just for your own satisfaction, but for your partner's as well.

Believe it or not, declining, hormone-driven sex actually creates the opportunity for greater intimacy. This can

Dr. Dorree Says:

Physically, you cannot compete with the younger version of yourself, so why try? Instead, you can take advantage of your declining hormones and slow down and experience something new. When it comes to true intimacy, that younger guy you used to be probably could not compete with you now.

take a little getting used to. The old "slam-bang, thank you, ma'am" approach is not especially conducive to conversations leading to connection, and it may have allowed you to have decades of sex without really exposing yourself or sharing much with your partner. Slowing down creates the time and space for you to relax and open up with another person. This is not typically something that every younger man finds appealing. But they don't know what they are missing, and now, challenging as it might be, you have the opportunity to find out.

Seven Male Myths about Sex

Male Myth #1: It's not sex unless you have intercourse.
(**False.** Sex is more than hitting the target's bull's eye).

Seven Male Myths about Sex *(cont'd)*

Male Myth #2: It's not sex unless you have an orgasm. (**False.** Sex is an attitude and self-image. An "I love you" qualifies as sex, as does a caring caress).

Male Myth #3: Sex is performance. You either succeed or fail. (**False.** Sex is a process, not a goal).

Male Myth #4: Men don't express feelings. (**False.** Sort of. Most men prefer to fix a problem rather than discuss it, but many will be open if you open the dialogue in a non-confrontational way).

Male Myth #5: All sexual feelings have an end goal. (**False.** Feelings are different from actions. Most men have feelings and fantasies that they don't always act on).

Male Myth #6: Men always have to initiate sex. (**False.** Each partner is equally responsible for starting the process).

Male Myth #7: Men can't have multiple orgasms. (**False.** With rest and relaxation, many men can come more than once).

Relationships: Stay, Go, or Grow?

QUESTION: *My wife and I have been together for twenty-three years. The kids are grown and the extra time we now have together is making it harder to ignore the fact that we just don't like each other all that much anymore. I am torn between relishing the idea of getting out of here and not wanting to lose something that took us years to create. What should I do?*

—JACK, 52

Many couples begin to reevaluate their relationships in midlife. Sometimes, only one party wants out, while the other has no idea that things are not going as well as they think. Often the woman is the first to voice her dissatisfaction, maybe even filing for divorce.

While women are quicker to file for divorce than men, husbands are more likely to stay unhappily married and have affairs, which may later lead to the end of their marriages. For some men, once the children are out of the house, it may be tempting to say, "The kids are gone, why not me too?" Interestingly, most marriages today do not end when an affair is discovered. (Couples are much more likely to split because of money issues than infidelity).

On the other hand, simply staying together after an affair does not mean the marriage has significantly improved. Maintaining a deeply satisfying intimate relationship is challenging at every age, and at midlife perhaps even more so. (For more on how to revive a boring relationship, please see Chapters 5 and 6.) But the happiness and health value of being in a good relationship can make the extra effort so worthwhile. In fact, a recent study by researchers at the University of Chicago and Johns Hopkins Bloomberg School of Public Health found that, compared to married people, those who are divorced or widowed have 20 percent more chronic health conditions, such as heart disease, diabetes, or cancer. They also have 23 percent more mobility limitations, such as trouble climbing stairs or walking a block. So divorce can be injurious to your physical and emotional health.

Both men and women need close connections with others, such as a mate, but a surprising myth buster for many is that studies show that men may need it even more. Women are more likely to connect with friends and community, while many men tend to isolate themselves from others, especially as they age. Older men who live alone do quite poorly, both physically and emotionally, and are at greater risk for illnesses, even suicide.

So even though women are more likely to be interested in improving the relationship, the effort required to create and maintain a good relationship may actually pay greater health and happiness returns for a man than for a woman.

Leaving your marriage or long-term partnership is always an option and can sometimes be a good idea, but why rush it? Now that the kids are gone and the two of you have more freedom than before, what harm would it do to experiment with some of the suggestions offered in the rest of this book before you call it quits? If you try putting a different effort into what is your known relationship and hit the jackpot because your relationship gets added buzz, you could be rewarded for your efforts for many, many years. But even with tons of effort, if you still come up empty, you know you've done your best and can leave with less internal push-and-pull.

Fantasies

Remember when former president Jimmy Carter admitted to having "lust in my heart," and the media had a heyday with his very common desire, but uncommonly expressed comment? It's perfectly normal and natural for men to fantasize about having sex with other women (or men or multiple partners in various combinations). After 50, this doesn't stop. If anything, after so many years of perhaps raising a family and dealing with the daily grind of life, older men are even more likely than younger men to think about sex with others, especially with a younger partner. And why not? Millions of years of evolution have arranged it so that we find young men and women in their physical prime especially sexually attractive. Unless you can no longer see, you will probably notice this fact wherever you go.

> **Dr. Dorree Says:**
>
> In all my years of practice, I've never known an older man who hasn't at least dreamed about having sex with a younger woman. Fantasy is not the same as action.

Feeling guilty about this can only add to your stress unnecessarily. Thinking is not doing. Fantasizing about anything with anyone is not cheating. Most men (and women) fantasize before and during sex. It can be a wonderful way to help you get turned-on and enhance sex, alone or with a partner.

Sometimes there are actions that *do* go beyond fantasy, but are not quite like having an affair. Take Jeffrey, for example. Married to Evelyn for eighteen years, he loves the lure of strip joints and lap dances. In truth, he'd really like to go a lot further and play around more. The only thing that stops him from having full-blown affairs with both women and men is his brain, not his desire. So he splits the difference and has his fringe flings. So far, he hasn't chosen to have intercourse with anyone other than his wife, even when he wants to. He just can't bring himself to risk hurting his wife and three children. At heart, he values family and lives with fantasies—and just a bit more.

Affairs

It's normal for a man's mind to wander to greener pastures on occasion—and sometimes, your penis may follow. Most men and women are serial monogamists, meaning they stay loyal to one person until they move on to their next intimate relationship. A significant minority have multiple lovers, often without their primary partners' knowledge. Men are more likely than women to have affairs, according to *The Monogamy Myth* by Peggy Vaughan (Newmarket Press, 2003), which estimates that 60 percent of men and 40 percent of women have extramarital affairs. An earlier study by the University of California puts the numbers much lower, at 24 percent of married men and 14 percent of married women.

Therapists generally believe the percentage of affairs outside marriage is much closer to those stated by Vaughan, because respondents aren't always forthcoming in self-reporting studies. According to a Time-CNN poll, 50 percent of Americans say President Clinton's adultery makes his moral standard "about the same as the average married man," which also suggests that the statistics are far higher.

Some wives seem to have an extra antenna when it comes to affairs. You may think you are getting away with it, but then all of a sudden she's on to you. Known affairs can put a tremendous strain on a relationship and can take a lot of work and time to heal, if they don't lead to divorce. So think before you leap. Only you can decide what is best for you in each situation.

If you do have an affair and want to remain in your original relationship, be aware that it can take its toll on your partnership and it will take effort and time to regain trust. You can also take heart in the knowledge that recent studies show that affairs, although challenging to recover from, do not break relationships up as much as some people may think. The trend is to stay together and forgive, or at least stay together and move on.

Fantasy or Infidelity?

In his mind, Raymond has never been unfaithful to his wife, although he always wanted to be. For years, he desperately wanted sex with other women. On business trips, Raymond was partial to visiting strip clubs and topless bars. One time, he paid for a lap dance and ejaculated inside his pants. The next time, Raymond got a lap dance and a blow job, which he felt was heavenly. He repeated this many times over the years of his marriage, but never went any further.

After every encounter, Raymond's penis became intensely itchy for a few days. It got so bad that he finally had his doctor check it out, but no physical cause could be found. He was "itching" to have an affair and his sexual encounters didn't help. Raymond had an itch he couldn't scratch—in more ways than one!

Interestingly, once he started wearing a condom during these excursions, the penis itching went away, so who knows, maybe it was something physical after all, like candida. Or maybe it was Raymond's thinking that changed with the condom. Perhaps he felt more at ease and responsible, and therefore less guilty. It's hard to know when it's mind over matter. The mind-body connection runs so deep.

For some people, lap dances and blow jobs with another person do constitute being unfaithful to their primary relationship, and they choose not to play that way. Other people have open marriages and accept that their partners may have multiple

> **Dr. Dorree Says:**
>
> I don't believe men are naturally monogamous. The psychology of evolution simply says this isn't so. It is a choice based on your personal morality and how you will feel in the morning.

sexual encounters, with or without them. Still other people may have emotional affairs, which often develop at places like work, that they wish could progress to the bedroom, but never do. Like most things involving sex, what you choose to do and how you feel about it is a personal matter between you and your partners.

Become a Condom Connoisseur

Whatever you do, use condoms. Sexually transmitted diseases are on the rise among men and women over 50. Few men really like using condoms, so it's worth spending some time finding the best one for you. As with purchasing a new top coat, try different brands and types: ultra thin condoms, ribbed condoms, latex, and polyurethane condoms—and even different sizes. Take your stash home and practice masturbating with what you've got. Use a lubricant, inside and out, if you find it helps. When you find the right match, keep one or several handy at all times. Unless you are in a long-term monogamous relationship, you may wind up saving your own life.

Great Sex Unzipped

QUESTION: *I understand that it's normal for sex to change as we age. How can I use what I have to enjoy the best sex possible for as long as possible?*

—RAJNI, 72

Like many things in life, from your muscles to your mind, you either use it or you lose it. In general, the more good sex you have now, the more good sex you can have later. Here are some time-tested tips for keeping it alive:

- Getting turned-on is good for you. Many men are visual and enjoy pornography. If Internet porn fits with your life, and your relationship with it is not addictive, pornographic websites can be a convenient visual resource.
- Fantasy is wonderful for your sex life, with or without a partner. Remember, thinking is not doing.
- Have sex when you are aroused, either alone or with a partner. The more often you do it (within reason), the better.
- Get a partner of your sexual preference. (If you don't have one, see Chapter 7 for ways to find someone.)
- Go slow and enjoy the moment. Slower sex is not only easier on you physically, it's also more intimate. Most women love it. You may find you love it, too.
- Exercise your pelvic floor muscles by doing Kegels. (Repeatedly tighten and release the muscles that would stop the flow of urine if you were peeing). This isotonic exercise helps men control ejaculation, and because no one knows you are doing it, it can be done anywhere, anytime, even at the bus stop.
- Good food and moderate exercise will help keep your weight down and your penis up. Don't cheat yourself out of a great second half of life with unhealthy habits that don't support you now or in the future.
- Don't compare yourself, your partner, and your sex life to what you see in porn videos. Those people are actors, their bodies do not represent the norm, and they don't behave like most adults. Fun to watch, but it isn't real-life.
- Have sex the way you like it, and teach it to your partner.
- Relax as much as possible. Stress is no friend of sex. Stress and anxiety interfere with performance, so worries about performance are self-fulfilling.

- Learn relaxation techniques (like yoga, meditation, bio-feedback, deep breathing) to quiet your thoughts for mind-blowing sex.
- Keep up with or start strength- and stamina-building exercises. They will help keep you healthy enough to be active in bed.
- Consider some of the Eastern sex arts discussed in Chapter 5.

How to Be the World's Best Lover

Back when the sex hormones of our youth were running the show, all we needed was a willing partner and we were off to the races. After 50, we have the luxury of slowing down and engaging our minds more. Sperm delivery is not the only goal. Learning how to extend the pleasure for both you and your partner can also be quite satisfying.

Given that the two of you do not share the same body and thoughts, great sex often involves communication, asking, and listening. We all tend to give what we want to get. This often does not work very well. Find out what your partner enjoys and learn how to do it. Study your partner's body and practice what she (or he) wants, like learning to play a fine violin. Show her or him how to do the same.

Be open to trying new things. Experiment and discover. No one is watching or keeping score. These experiments and experiences are just for the two of you.

Consider extending foreplay for as long as possible. Slow down and enjoy each sensation. Women generally need a little more time than men to "warm up," and the longer ramp-up can heighten your pleasure as well.

While great sex can happen because of a spontaneous moment or an unplanned new position, planning ahead can be fun, as well as helpful for making it happen in today's busy world. Regular "date nights," sex at unusual times (such as afternoon delights), scheduled sex times, and trips away together, short or long, all give you and your partner something to look forward to—time that is entirely for your mutual pleasure.

Seven Things Women Wish Men Knew About Sex

1. Chivalry is not dead. Despite being equals, women still appreciate men who hold the door, pull out the chair, and treat them with respect.
2. Sex starts long before bed. A hug by the sink, a kiss on the neck on the way to work, holding hands at the movies, and other affectionate touching can get a woman more in the mood. Even helping around the house so she can have some downtime is foreplay for many!
3. Make your woman feel desirable. You may have seen her naked a thousand times before, but each time is a privilege and an opportunity to show her that she still turns you on.
4. A slow hand is a turn-on. An occasional firecracker quickie is fine, but most women like a slow buildup to a big bonfire.
5. Learn what your lover likes, not just what you think she likes. Ask, learn, and practice.
6. Pillow talk is sexy. Few things turn a woman on more than hearing her lover open up about something intimate. A little conversation afterward is comforting, too. Rolling over and going right to sleep is almost always a bummer.

Seven Things Women Wish Men Knew About Sex (cont'd)

7. Clean is sexy! If you work in the oil fields all day, please take a shower before bed.

Am I Too Old for Sex?

You're never too old for sex! Your marvelous sex organs may respond more slowly or differently than when you were a kid, but they never wear out. In fact, having regular sex is excellent for your health at every age, and especially good for you later in life.

Learning how to have great sex after 50 often means learning how to have sex differently than when you were a young man. It may take new communication techniques you've never tried. It may mean taking a chance on dating again, or for the first time. And even if you have health problems that slow you down, there are many creative ways to learn how to enjoy sex anyway. For a while, all these changes may make you feel strange, even vulnerable. The key to forever-sex is to customize your performance power with new tools and skills that will bring you a lifetime of pleasure.

Remember, guys, at every age and stage you're still the main man and lovers still want you!

FIVE

BETWEEN THE SHEETS
Great Sex from 50 to 100

Want to have great sex for the rest of your life? Want to have the kind of sex that is actually fun (not just a favor for your mate or to prove your potency), that feels great to the body you have now, and that adds genuine intimacy and deep satisfaction to your years?

We know that sex naturally changes in midlife and beyond. What will be your particular version of sex next? So many things are not knowable or controllable in life, but how you choose to be sexual now and in the future (within your physical limits) really is up to you. With or without a partner, sex can be an exciting element of your life; it can keep your juices flowing and your energy up; it can make you smile and add years to your life. There are many ways you may not have thought of yet to make your life more sexually user-friendly and to make sex with the body you have today the best it has ever been since you passed puberty.

Seems unlikely? See what you think after you check out

121

some of these real-life sex secrets for ages 50 to 100. No matter what your age and situation, there just might be something here that can knock your socks off.

Forget Your Sun Sign—What's Your Sex Style?

QUESTION: *This might sound nutty, but my husband and I love to tickle each other in bed until we both feel turned-on and ready for sex. Are we weird?*

—KAREN, 63

Actually, you're lucky you both like the same thing and have found a fun way to get your sexual energies flowing. Isn't it wonderful that the same things turn you on, and if tickling makes you smile, how delightful. No one is watching or passing judgment on what turns you on behind closed doors. Even if this has been your foreplay style for years, be aware that people do grow and change over time. Be sensitive to adapting your style if one of you no longer finds this fun. The happiest couples don't expect things never to change; they make the effort to evolve together.

Individuals and couples often develop their own sex styles that partially reflect their personalities and relationships. Every sex style is good if you both enjoy it and it leads to satisfying sex. Experimenting with another style once in a while can be exciting, too. Like food, variety really does add spice to life. Occasionally, a rigid sex style can block you from experiencing other kinds of lovemaking. Remember, no individual or couple is ever all one style, but most do have preferences or patterns. Which one are you?

Funny sex. You laugh and tease one another in bed. For you, foreplay and sex are all about having fun together. Potential blind spot: you might be missing out on the more relaxed and intimate side of sex.

Angry sex. You make love even when you're ticked off at each other, or maybe right after a big blowup. This sex style can be healing, as long as you make sure that your problems are eventually talked about and resolved. Potential blind spot: when do you get a chance to make love without war first?

Lusty sex. This style can be full of wicked and flirty looks at each other, a passionate kiss in the grocery store when no one is looking, an unexpected quickie, and the joy of having sex just for the sake of sex. Potential blind spot: lusty sex alone sometimes becomes a way to avoid emotional intimacy and vulnerability.

Tender sex. You love gentle, romantic, healing sex that may involve soothing massage, light touches, candlelight, soft music, sharing secrets, and ministering to each another. Potential blind spot: where's the heat?

Fantasy sex. Your adventuresome spirit is to be envied by many. Role-playing, costumes, fetishes, images (alone or shared) provide saucy spice. Potential blind spot: make sure your real lover remains in the picture.

Comfort sex. Just another ho-hum, tired-at-the-end-of-the-day roll in the hay. You snuggle next to each other, some caressing starts, maybe there's intercourse, maybe not. You feel connected and relaxed before falling asleep. Potential blind spot: Comfort patterns are easy to get into and difficult to leave. Keep some reserve energy for times of desire and passion.

Accommodating sex. He/she wants sex and you go along.

You're not that into it at first, but can lie back (or just relax) and enjoy it if your partner initiates and does most of the "work." Sometimes, pleasing a horny partner is generous. Potential blind spot: could become a habit unless you make sure the favor is returned and you still have times of mutual passion.

Wild-side sex. You go for new sex toys, whips, chains, ceiling hooks, films, pornography, and erotic books. Potential blind spot: make sure your body can twist like a pretzel, and ask yourself if you still have desire even without all the extra bells and whistles.

Tantric or Kama Sutra sex. You both breathe deeply and mutually expand your sexual (and possibly even spiritual) experiences by focusing on the process rather than only on the end goal. Potential blind spot: Are you gaining a new, passionate experience or losing your fire? Take a pass on the self-criticism if this kind of sex turns out not to be your thing.

Making Love When You Don't Love Your Body

QUESTION: *My husband never mentions my weight and sagging breasts, but I feel like an old, fat cow. How am I ever going to feel sexy again?*

—TRACEY, 58

Your body has changed and probably, if you're like most Americans, many parts have drooped. There is no reason to hide in the closet or get dressed in the bathroom. Your partner's body has probably drooped as well. Boobs sag, tummies pop, butts and thighs jiggle, and wrinkles appear (unless you live in a cosmetic surgeon's office, they will appear even if you

exercise). If you were a bit chubby
before, you're probably even heavier
now. People who are on the slim side
develop angles instead of curves and
have bony knobs and bumps that
never existed before. Body types are

Dr. Dorree Says:

Every inch of your body
is a miracle. Sexy is not a
body size or shape—it's
a frame of mind.

as varied as people; we age differently but all bodies do change.

What are you going to do, dislike yourself for the next forty
years? That's a long time to be miserable. How about a new
way of looking at yourself that could be a lot more fun for you
(and probably for your partner, too)?

This is your beautiful body, the one that is keeping you alive
right this minute and letting you enjoy life. This is the body that
gave you children, if you have any, the one that got you to work
every day for many years, that got you through countless bouts
of colds and flu and who knows what else, and that helped you
survive for the last fifty or more years and got you here today.

Love your body, enjoy it, and get to know it. Share it with your
partner and get to know his or her body. If you've never looked
at your vagina, take out a mirror and look. Feel comfortable
enough to have your partner look, too, if he or she is interested.
One of the joys of getting older (hopefully) is you have time to
pay attention to some things that you once took for granted—
like your marvelous body. Toss out those airbrushed, model-
perfect magazine images in your mind, and start hanging out
with people who look more like you and share your interests and
reality. Eat well, live well, be physically active, and focus on something you like about yourself and you've been too shy to pay
attention to. Change your attitude about who you are and how
sexy you can be. We bet your body image will change, as well.

Touch and Be Touched

Touch is the elixir and essence of sex as we age. Any kind of nurturing touch, with clothes on or off, can increase sexual desire. Know your own special erotic spots and those of your partner: breasts, back, toes, elbows, thighs, nape of the neck, whatever turns you on. Take charge of your own sexuality. The more you know about your body (and your partner's), the better your experience will be. The more you can share about your knowledge of yourself with your partner, the better sex will be.

Dr. Dorree Says:

Remember, your partner shares your bed but not your head; please tell her or him what you like.

If you don't fully know what you like, now is a good time to find out. Try different ways of touching yourself or ask your partner to explore with you. Masturbation is always good, especially if you haven't had an orgasm in a while and want to "wake yourself up." Even if you know what you like, masturbation can help you fine-tune the touch you like best.

Mutual masturbation can be great fun, too. Clitoral stimulation by your partner can work wonders. When it's good, it's very, very good, but when it's bad . . . well, you know the rest. Learn what pleases your clitoris and teach it to your partner. Depending on your comfort zone, you can say it verbally ("a little harder, a little to the right") or nonverbally through touch (such as guiding your partner's hand). Penises can be pleasured in as many ways as there are men. Masturbation teaches you what turns you on, and then you can show your partner what to do.

Go with the Flow

Every day you are a new person, so certainly after many years together, you and your partner have changed quite a bit. Be aware of what you like now and what your partner may now prefer.

Women, for example, may find that their once-sensitive nipples are often less so now due to hormonal changes, and in a few cases they may be more sensitive. Do you like your breasts and nipples touched? If so, what ways are best? Find out and tell your partner.

Men will often have softer or less consistently hard erections, which is perfectly normal. Instead of strong, forceful ejaculations, some men find that, although their ejaculations are gentler, they can last longer. Enjoy your new body and possibilities. What you lose in terms of intensity, you gain in a different kind of experience, duration, and with sufficient rest, repetitive power. Sex changes, and its new ways can feel better than before.

With age, most people are responsive to a gentler touch. Sudden or strong movements can be startling or even scary. Touch and enjoy full-body contact until you want something more. When we were young, we could go from zero to sixty miles per hour very fast, and then could easily do it again. These days, there's less of a hurry. Slow down and enjoy the experience. (Remember that song "Slow Hand," sung by the Pointer Sisters, Conway Twitty, and others?)

Hugging and cuddling are types of touch that many people adore. But some do not. Frequently, one partner wants more hugging than the other. Be aware of which one of you wants to withdraw first or prefers to continue. Hugs, like most of what goes into sex, are often simply not paid attention to. With awareness of each person's preferences, you can avoid building feelings of abandonment or suffocation, and instead, meet somewhere in a satisfying middle. Hugging, even when not overtly sexual, is part of foreplay, even if it's hours or days away from when you actually have intercourse.

Men, please take note: foreplay is not a recipe (eight minutes of this, five minutes of that) or a let's-get-it-over-with toll bridge to the rest of sex. Women, please understand: foreplay contains the word "play" for a reason; make it fun and enjoyable for yourself and your partner, not something you have to do to get him hard enough and you wet enough for intercourse. Foreplay should not be a chore for either party. If it is, it's probably time for something new, or perhaps your relationship needs a sex tune-up (see Chapter 6).

If you use lubricants, vibrators, vaginal inserts, cock rings, or any other toys (see Chapter 9), keep them handy, maybe in a velvet box. These toys can be the jewels of your older years (and may help keep your own jewels alive).

Speak Up!

Sex, as with all of life, requires negotiation. If any part of sex is unpleasant, terribly boring, or has become something you want to avoid, revisiting both your attitude and the mechanics can have a dramatic impact on your sex life. Great lovers know how to take their time and pay attention to small communication cues. One of the luxurious benefits of added years is, although the body may get tired more easily, the upside is you actually have more time to explore the small pleasures in and out of bed that turn you and your partner on.

All this takes speaking up. Embarrassment, especially at our age, though common, is really a waste of time. Look for communication tips and ideas in Chapter 6. If talking about what you like is too difficult, you can show your partner with actions, or read a sex book together, go to a movie, go to a museum, take a walk, and talk about what you have seen. If people are too shy to speak directly, they can use what's around them to make slow inroads to creative nonverbal communication.

The Fine Art of Kissing

QUESTION: *My boyfriend is really sweet and sex has been pretty good, but I don't like the way he kisses. Is there anything I can do?*

—CORA, 62

You know how "they" keep telling you not to try to change someone, to just love them as they are? Well, that's mostly true, but who says you can't teach an old kisser some new tricks? In many ways, we do teach partners (and they teach us) to make love in a new way that is a melding of the two.

How about telling your boyfriend that you love having sex with him and you'd like to make it even better by trying new ways to kiss? Maybe make it a game and try a new kind of kissing each day. Or ask him to experiment with changing one particular thing, such as holding his breath or keeping his lips too rigid. The key here is relaxed experimentation and feedback. Talk about what you each like. For example, do you know if your boyfriend likes the way *you* kiss?

After touching, kissing is high on the list of what makes sex mysteriously work. Whether it's your first kiss ever or your last kiss with your current love, kissing can be magical. Or it can become boring and routine. There are a million good ways to kiss. With the passing years, why stay with the same old, same old? Maybe you've always preferred a peck on the cheek, or perhaps deep, tongue "French" kissing got lost along the way while you were raising children or chasing a career. Many times, especially in long-term relationships, people can forget how much they used to like kissing and may become complacent lovers. There may be other reasons, as well. For some people, kissing may be more intimate than intercourse and they are holding themselves back from feeling too vulnerable.

It's never too late to change how you kiss. Play with kissing to see what works for you—pecks, deep soul-kissing, the quickie, butterfly kiss—what do you like? If you always kiss in just one or two ways, try something new and see what happens!

Lose Your Mind, Come to Your Senses

One of the silver linings of declining sex hormones for both men and women is that the less intense focus on the genitals means you can more fully focus on the sensations of your entire body and all your senses. Enjoying your skin (your biggest sex organ) and all your senses (taste, touch, smell, sight, and hearing) can be like exploring a playground.

If you are accustomed to keeping your eyes closed during sex, try opening them and looking at your partner. Or close them, if that's new for you, and delve deeply inside yourself for a change. Listen to each other's breath and to the other sounds of passion. Taste yourself and each other. And enjoy the many fragrances of being close. Probably the most undervalued sense, smell, plays a greater role in attraction and bonding than you may know. Smell helps people fall in love, and surprisingly, research shows that liking your partner's smell is one of the most reliable predictors of the longevity of the relationship.

Quieting your mind and immersing yourself in all the sensations of the body can make sex all the more wonderful. Try to let go, relax, and be comfortable with whatever you (or you and your partner) do.

Dr. Dorree Says:

Like enjoying a satisfying meal, sex doesn't have to be gourmet fare each and every time for it to be sustaining and satisfying.

Remember, there needn't be any grades or judgments involved, just your own experience of okay, good, or great sex.

Stalking the Illusive Orgasm

QUESTION: *I've been married for thirty-two years and have four grown children. I've had sex countless times in my life but I've never had an orgasm. What's wrong with me?*

—JANE, 57

Some people just never have orgasms and they come to accept that. If you are one of those people, there may be nothing at all wrong with you. On the other hand, there may be something you can do if you want to have an orgasm. If you can climax while masturbating, but not during intercourse, then the issue is learning how to repeat that with your partner. Have you been too shy to talk about it or show him what you enjoy? Satisfying sex with another person, especially with someone you share a long-term commitment with, takes communication (verbal and nonverbal), negotiation (sex changes as we change), and most of all, courage! None of us are getting any younger. If this is an experience you want to have, now could be a great time to begin actively pursuing it.

If you have never experienced an orgasm, even by yourself, and want that to change, the key is to masturbate. Choose times when your privacy won't be interrupted and perhaps experiment with a vibrator or using water pressure in the tub or shower. Be patient and persistent. For added stimulation, maybe try reading some erotic literature or watching pornography geared for women. If unwanted feelings arise, keep a journal nearby to record them. And consider seeking help from a counselor if memories of adult or childhood trauma or abuse are getting in your way. Once you clear what's blocking you and learn how to wake up your body, that illusive orgasm you seek might well become a regular part of your love life.

If you are one of those who have never been orgasmic, no matter what you do, it may never happen. Sometimes hormones are the reason, or psychological blocks, or a host of other possibilities. So what? You are fine just as you are. Remember sex is more than penetration and certainly more than a few quick muscle contractions at the end. In fact, many who espouse India's version of tantric sex believe focusing on orgasm as the end goal diminishes the opportunity for total body enjoyment. So whether or not you are orgasmic, enjoy every bodily sensation.

Swapping the "Shopping List" Sex for Something Steamier

Ladies, do you find yourself thinking about the laundry or what to pick up at the store for dinner during sex? This is perfectly normal for some women and is not a reflection of how much you care about your partner or how good you are in bed. It's natural for some woman (and even some men) to think about nonsexy things at the start of sex and maybe right in the middle, as well.

What can we do about this? If it doesn't bother you, don't do a thing! No one knows what you are thinking about, and after a few minutes you will probably be focusing on more physical pleasures. But if it does bother you and you'd like to trade in your shopping-list mind chatter for something more delightful, how about taking a fun sexual fantasy out for a spin?

Since your mind is already wandering, what's the harm? Most people have sexual fantasies and most people feel guilty about it, unnecessarily. Men, if they are willing to be honest, often fantasize scenes that you might see in porn movies (with the woman in high heels, stockings, white pearls, and nothing more, her head thrown back in squeals of sexual ecstasy). Most women feel objectified by such a scenario, but if you can understand that you are giving your man pleasure, this can be a turn on for you, too. Woman tend to have a wide variety of sexual fantasies, from complex story lines to base rape scenes to forbidden sex with someone they dare not approach in real life. In fact, women tend to love reading erotica. These sexy stories don't have to stay in your head only; you can read them aloud or retell them to your partner after you read them.

If you want to really turn up the heat, consider sharing your hottest sexual fantasy with your partner and ask to hear his or hers. It can be a turn-on to share fantasies and then wonder about what your partner might be thinking about as you make love. You can even use props and costumes to act out a fantasy, if you feel so inclined.

Some Like It Hot

If the brain is the most powerful sex organ, surely fantasy is one of its most potent energizers. Allow yourself the pleasure of fantasizing before and during sex. You can keep these sexy thoughts entirely private, dare to share them with your partner as a turn-on, or even boldly experiment with enacting some of them, if you are both agreeable.

Richard, 62, and Karen, 59, tried acting out a shared fantasy and it rocked their sex life. After nearly three decades of marriage, things had gotten pretty boring in bed. Both partners fantasized during sex, as many men and women often do. Then one day, Karen took the lead by revealing one of her "operating room" fantasies to Richard as they were making love, which greatly turned them both on. Sex was so good that night, Karen decided to take it a step further and secretly purchased a sexy nurse's uniform online.

The day it came in the mail, Karen put on the outfit under her usual bathrobe. Later, when the couple was getting ready for bed, Karen dropped her old robe to the floor and ordered Richard to "lie down on the operating table." Though at first embarrassed and a bit in shock, her husband quickly obeyed as his nurse draped him (even his face) with a sheet, exposing only his penis. She then preformed an "operation" on him involving a silk scarf, ice, and whipped cream. A strap-on vibrator under her costume added to Karen's building passion. When her patient was close to climax, she dropped her vibrator, straddled her husband, and they both exploded in orgasm together. It was one of the best sexual experiences of their lives.

Experiment with New Sex Positions

QUESTION: *I'm getting tired of making love in the missionary position, but I'm not the kind of guy who knows a lot about sex. What else can we comfortably do at our age?*

—MARK, 76

"At our age" we can do a whole lot! If sex is getting boring or your genitals need more encouragement, this can be the time of life to be more creative and adventuresome. If an old position no longer works as well for you, there are many other ways to *do it*.

Because different sex positions don't normally come up in conversation at a cocktail party or even with your best friend, turning to books or Internet sites can be a great resource: you know the old adage that "a picture is worth a thousand words." But remember, even if you used to be able to twist your body like a pretzel, unless you are in amazing shape today, you are probably salted and peppered with aches and pains and aren't as flexible as you once were. As you move into new terrain, be gentle with yourself and don't try anything that can hurt.

Proceed with caution, as well, when going online. Have a spam blocker and a mechanism to clear your computer's history. Many people are afraid to go to the Web for sex information—such as new positions—because it looks like they're going after porn material. There is a difference. Do stay away from the porn sites or they will surely not stay away from you. However, there are many informational sites out there, such as Dr. Dorree's FiftyandFurthermore.com, that are entirely legitimate.

Some picture books and websites with positions for older people are very unrealistic. Most people couldn't do some of their suggested positions even if they were 20! How many women can stretch their legs way over their heads, and how many men can carry on like Tarzan? After 50, most of us want comfortable positions. If missionary style has been your thing for years and doesn't work for you anymore (or is just plain boring), you can add spice to your sex life by experimenting with some of the following new moves.

Woman on top, facing forward. This is a great change from the man-on-top missionary style. The woman sits straddling her partner, and after he becomes hard or she helps him become stiff enough for penetration, she can insert his penis inside her. They can both use their hands freely to caress, pinch, or massage themselves and/or each other. She can use any motion she wants: up and down, round and round, at any speed she desires. The lovely shift that this position offers is that a man can surrender and a woman can feel in control.

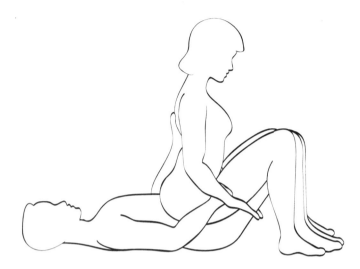

Woman on top, facing backward. If you are self-conscious about your tummy or other body parts, this position gives you some privacy while giving both of you the possibility for deep penetration, provided the man can sustain a firm enough erection. At the same time, her lover can caress her often neglected back and buttocks, and the women can swirl, curve, do figure eights with her hips, and experiment with various circular and up-and-down motions. With his feet firmly planted on the bed or floor (but no rug burns please), she can use his knees for support. This is also a great position for adding a basic vibrator or even a rabbit (see Chapter 9). The man can even caress her perineum and/or anus, or insert a finger or two or a sex toy in her anus.

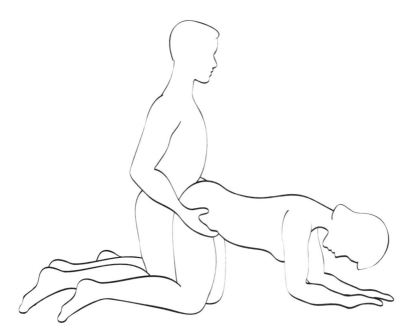

Rear entry of the vagina. With the man on his knees behind his partner, the woman rests on both elbows and knees, "doggy style," in front of him. Many couples find this their most primal and animalistic position. With age and weight gain, this position can allow a man to freely use his hands to stimulate the woman's clitoris, or if he is tall enough, he can bend over and nibble her neck. A pillow propped under the woman can free up her hands to caress her breasts or finger her clitoris or her partner's testes. The woman must be careful not to overly arch her back to avoid injury. The other disadvantage to this position is that it doesn't permit face-to-face contact for a full-frontal connection. But the joys of a change of pace can outweigh potential negatives.

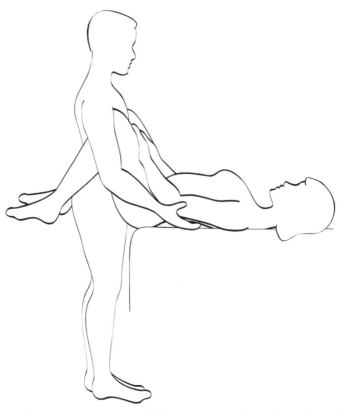

Standing intercourse. The man stands at the edge of the bed and the women lies on her back with her bottom as close as possible to her partner and her legs spread. This is a wonderful position when there is a significant height difference between the partners. Many men also enjoy the freedom of being able to thrust without worrying about a bad back. If you're on a bed, or perhaps even some place out of the norm, like a table or a chair, and there's a wall to lean on, so much the better. It's also easier for many women who find their bodies don't readily curve into an acrobatic C-shape. He can hold her legs up at almost any angle that is mutually comfortable. You can adjust the height of the bed to suit your needs (see Chapter 6).

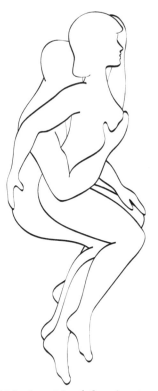

Spooning/side-by-side. After beginning the rear-entry position, both partners then gently flop over onto their sides without disengaging. With added years, almost any position that
gives added comfort, takes less energy, and doesn't require
acrobatic ability, can be very welcome.

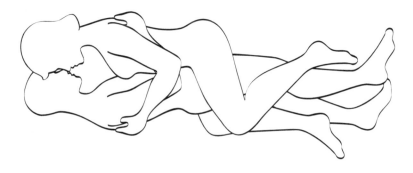

Face-to-face, side-by-side. This gives total body access, intimacy, and except for getting one's legs out of the way of your genitals, can become a favorite, even over the standard missionary position. This may be the easiest position of all as it requires the least acrobatics. You simply lie down, face each other, and hug. Then help your genitals participate as well.

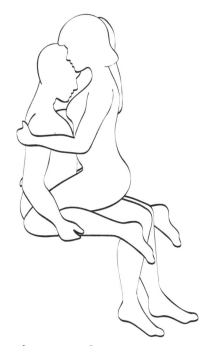

Sitting in a chair. A variety of sitting positions may be worth exploring, especially when one partner has limited mobility (perhaps wheelchair-bound) or has a bad back or joint pains.

The permutations are endless. Be creative. There are many more position possibilities to try. Props can be a welcome addition, especially for aching joints or a vulnerable back. Use a pillow or two, and see what new angles you can find. Some couples even like to add a mirror above or to the side of the bed. It can be a simple way to double the visual fun. Some people like to set up a video camera and take their own home movies. But be careful about

Dr. Dorree Says:

Let your imagination be your guide. For more ideas, you can explore pictures of every kind in books, films, and online, together or alone, and see what appeals to you.

where you keep these very personal recordings. Remember what happened to Pamela Anderson and so many others.

Too Shy for Sexually Explicit Books and Websites?

If you are among the many people who just can't bring themselves to look at explicit sex books and websites with your partner or even by yourself, here's a fun and classy alternative. Become an art connoisseur! Many cultures have a tradition of depicting sexual positions through fine art. Japanese and Chinese works of art are well respected for their erotica and many Indian temples are adorned with every sexual pose of the *Kama Sutra*. You can visit museums, peruse tasteful art books and websites, or even travel to see some of the art originals as part of a sexy vacation. And if you find some works of art particularly enthralling, a framed print or two on your bedroom wall might make a stimulating addition.

Oral Sex

For those who love it, oral sex can last a lifetime because it's fun, demands relatively little energy, and requires no high-flying acrobatics. If you've been intrigued but resistant, this could be a good time to see what you've been missing. Try it, you might like it! However, if it's never been your thing, it may never be appealing to you, which is fine. No matter. This is *your* sex life, not a checklist of other people's expectations you have to complete.

If you used to like oral sex years ago but haven't done it in a while, try going back to some old techniques that you've put on the shelf, even if you can't remember why. If you are diving in for the first time, or you want to expand your repertoire, start with gently kissing your partner's thighs, vulva, testicles; then move toward the genitals and add tongue, if you feel so inclined. Try experimenting with various ways of kissing, licking, and sucking. A creative combination of touching, mutual masturbation, sex toys, and oral sex can be so satisfying and exciting that you may skip intercourse all together.

Anal Sex

QUESTION: *My partner has been trying for months to convince me to have anal sex with him, which he says I am going to love. I've never tried it before and I am afraid it might hurt. What should I do?*

—MAGGIE ROSE, 59

If you don't want to try something, you certainly don't have to. On the other hand, it can be useful in life to have an open mind and at least consider something new. Some people like to be aroused or have orgasms from anal play, or from penile and vaginal play plus anal stimulation, with or without penetration. It's all good as long as you like it, your partner likes it, and no one gets hurts.

If you want to give this a try, you can start with gentle touching of the anus, perhaps with a neutral lubricant designed for this purpose. If you enjoy this and want to experiment further, you can try slowly inserting a finger tip (yours or his, with the nail well-trimmed) into the anus. A relaxed anus is capable of expanding and accepting a finger, dildo, or penis. Most people who engage in anal sex thoroughly enjoy it. Anything that hurts or feels uncomfortable can and should be immediately curtailed.

If this is something you'd like to try, here are some tips for first-timers.

- Discuss it ahead of time and agree on what you will and won't do. This is supposed to be pleasurable.
- Check your brain for any lingering myths that body parts are not supposed to be for fun. Your entire body belongs to you to enjoy as you please.
- Take a bath or shower first if you feel self-conscious about hygiene.
- Lubricate. Always err on the side of being extra wet. It feels good and prevents irritation or pain.
- Proceed gently. Anal tissues need time to expand to accommodate whatever enters. If it hurts or feels bad in any way, stop for a while and maybe try again with something smaller, like a finger.
- Give feedback about what you like and don't like. Remember to breathe and to bear down. People tend to hold their breath when anxious or in pain, constricting muscles that could otherwise easily relax and expand.
- Keep vibrators and sex toys clean and dry after each use. (Condoms make great sex toy covers). Consider putting a towel over your bed sheet as it is easier to wash (unless, of course, you are spontaneously bending over a chair, kitchen counter, or other creative place).
- Wash penis and sex toys before entering another orifice.

The one thing you never want to do or let your partner do is use any kind of anal desensitizer. The anus is fine for sex play and has delicate membranes of its own. Anything shoved up the rectum too quickly or anything inserted that may be too large can tear these delicate tissues. There is no reason to ever numb the anus. The nerve endings there function on many levels and help you have pleasurable sensations and slowly feel your way toward pleasure, not pain.

Tantric Sex, Kundalini, and the Kama Sutra

A growing number of older Americans are practicing sex techniques and philosophies from other cultures. In the U.S., sex is often promoted as a young person's sport—fast, competitive, and not too deeply felt. Ancient cultures, particularly many Eastern ones, such as in China, Japan, and India, have well-documented histories indicating that they have a broader view of sex. They see sex as something human beings can freely experience throughout their lifetimes that can also be a pathway to deeper experiences one can't usually reach in everyday life.

These sexual practices include tantric, kundalini, and *Kama Sutra* sex, as well as conscious breathing techniques to amplify the sexual experience. The basic idea behind all these approaches is that slowing down and taking your time with sex can be as sexy and fulfilling as the final orgasm, and perhaps even more so.

Practitioners of tantric sex, for example, find it blissful to have intercourse for prolonged minutes—some claim even hours—without having orgasm. For these lovers, it's the connection that counts. This method of intimacy focuses on an increased spiritual awareness and erotic energy. It can be practiced alone, but most often involves a lover. Think of tantric sexual connection as a dance with no beginning or end. There is no set foreplay and no orgasmic goal, only the union of present moment. Lovemaking becomes a process that is meditative, expressive, and intimate. With tantric sex, lovers learn how to extend the peak of their sexual ecstasy so that women *and* men can experience several orgasms in a single sexual encounter. Tantric sex takes patience, practice, commitment, and requires learning some basic breathing techniques, gentle stroking, and often involves gazing into each other's open eyes. Proponents of tantric sex consider it a wondrous opportunity for those no longer driven by the raging hormones of their youth. When partners have love, trust, and mutual respect, the magic of tantric sex is available to couples of all ages and levels of sexual experience. Obviously tantric's basic premise, which originates from both ancient Hindu and Buddhist practices, is very different from standard intercourse with orgasm as the ultimate goal. There's no rush to the finish line and the experience offers opportunity for intimacy no matter how rusty your parts are or how well everything else may be functioning. In fact, it is primarily the male partner who learns to delay orgasm by using PC muscles, the same group of muscles that one uses to stop urinating. It is a devotional expression of caring, in which sex can be a sacred part—and lots of fun, too!

The theory behind kundalini sex is that sexual energy is coiled like a metaphorical snake at the base of the spine, and with sexual arousal it starts to rise to higher levels, passing through the chakras (seven body points of deep, profound energy). Researchers of kundalini energy have mapped what happens in the brain during sexual arousal. Using Kirlian photography that changes color when exposed to different frequencies of energy, Western researchers have scientifically mapped what Eastern drawings have depicted for millennia. Energy ascends up the spine and approaches the brain as sexual feelings become stronger and stronger. When it reaches the crown of the head, in most people, the energy reverses and takes a downward course seeking release through the genitals as an orgasm.

Kama Sutra is an ancient Indian text and visual guide to sexual positions that hasn't changed in centuries and is still very useful today. If you aren't too shy to ask for it, you can even find the *Kama Sutra* in a video guide form. You can also look it up on the Internet to see the various positions. (But remember, stay away from porn sites.)

Sting Gets Real

Rock-star musician Sting and his activist wife, Trudie Styler, both over 50, are well-known advocates of tantric sex and credit their fulfilling sex life together to this ancient art. After much joking back and forth with a reporter about the general claim that some practitioners of tantric sex can go at it for many, many hours at a time, Sting finally set the record straight. Sure, we have sex for as long as eight hours, he said, if you include "dinner and a movie, followed by four hours of begging!"

Sex Therapy

If learning all this new sex stuff seems daunting, consider getting the equivalent of a coach. Some people prefer a relationship expert or couple's therapist, others try sex therapy to help break old patterns and learn new ones.

How to choose? Many people call themselves experts. As in any field, there are many phonies as well as pros. Don't be embarrassed to ask knowledgeable and trusted friends, your physician, clergyperson, local university, or hospital for a referral. Check with the American Association for Marriage and Family Therapy (AAMFT), American Association of Sexuality Educators Counselors and Therapists (AASECT), American Psychological Association, or other professional organizations listed in our reference section. When you get to the therapist's office, trust your gut. Does this person seem like he or she even has sex, or can help other people enjoy it more?

A good sex therapist will help you identify what to work on and give you exercises and techniques to practice at home, with or without a partner. (This is one time that homework, though perhaps a bit anxiety-producing, can be fun.) Like a good coach, a good sex therapist will help you develop your natural talents and help you make them just that much better. While therapist styles may differ, any sex therapist should be able to help you feel comfortable in their office, talk freely about your issues, explore intimacy barriers, and learn about sex positions (such as those mentioned in this chapter) and ways to pleasure yourself and your partner. Your therapist should be able to answer just about all your questions and even some you didn't know you wanted to ask. Issues that may be addressed by a sex therapist include:

- Are you able to tell your partner (or even admit to yourself) what you feel or want?
- Do your genitals function the way you expect them to?
- Do you lack libido?
- Do you carry messages from your past that persist in keeping you from trying anything sexually new?
- Do you have a secret sexual wish that you've never told your partner?

Really Senior Sex

The biggest sex secret of those over 50 is the fact that men and women in their 70s, 80s, and beyond still enjoy sex. Most people under 50 have no idea this is true and may even bristle at the mere thought of older people having intercourse. (Interestingly, even people who work in nursing homes have a hard time facing the fact that older people still "do it," especially if they themselves are under age 50.) Maybe we felt the same way when we were younger, but now that we are older, it's time to see this fact as the truly good news that it is. Sex lasts forever!

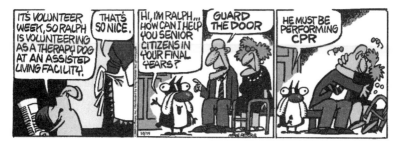

The great thing about senior sex is that, like CPR, it really can save lives.

What is the secret to really sizzling, senior sex? Clearly, it's not sex hormones. Few people over 50, and even fewer over 70, get aroused simply by hormonal desire alone. As sex hormones lose their zip, intercourse becomes less of a must-have goal, and sensuality can blossom. This means that keeping the connection between you alive is key to great sex in the later years (see Chapter 6 for ways to stay close in a long-term relationship). Communication, vulnerability, experimentation, creativity, and awareness of your own desires and comfort zones become more important than ever, the older we become. While the physical body may not be as limber as it used to be, there are still many ways to have great sex. Here's what seniors say helps the most.

- Stay or become good friends. Besides the sex, the side benefits are well worth it.
- Snuggle, hug, kiss, massage, and caress. It all helps get you in the mood.
- Don't rush. Allow excitement to build.
- Communicate. Communicate. Communicate (see Chapter 6). The more you talk to each another, the easier it is for your partner to know what you feel and desire. Plus, talking about sex can be a turn-on. Don't be shy, be direct.
- If talking is just too difficult for you, showing can work, too.
- Explore and be creative. Adapt to the changing needs of your bodies.
- Stay healthy and fit. It's sexier. Eat a balanced diet that includes lots of fruits and vegetables. Limit alcohol, quit smoking, and go for walks. Be aware that some illnesses and many medications can interfere with sexual desire and functioning (see Chapter 8).

For people who are well into their 80s and 90s, sex can evolve into something quite beautiful and rare—a combination of love, physical sensation, sensual play, generosity, nurturing, and self-expression that no pre-50 youngster could ever manage. People who take the time and effort to develop this kind of lovemaking over many years are truly our mentors as we each blaze our own trails into our new sexuality after 50.

A Sexy Great-Grandma

At 87, Leanne still works a few hours every day in her family's business, still drives her own car, still buys her own groceries, and yes, she still has sex. The mother of two and former nurse still can't quite bring herself to say the word "vagina," and she's never looked at her own genitals with a mirror, but she did discover a vibrator about ten years ago, which she uses only under the covers with the lights off, and she still enjoys having an orgasm "every once in a while," with or without her husband.

Amazing, after sixty years of marriage, through so many good times and bad, Leanne says her heart still sometimes skips a beat when her lover walks into the room. When asked how in the world she managed to stay with and have sex with the same man for so many years, Leanne winks with a knowing smile and answers, "Who says he's the same man?"

SIX

OH, NO! WHERE DID MY LOVER GO?
Great Sex in a Long-Term Relationship

If your relationship is always picture-perfect and sex is always stellar, skip this chapter. For the rest of us, let's get real. No matter how much we may love our partners, the road can be bumpy at times and sex in a long-term relationship can get pretty boring. Maybe there was a time when you couldn't keep your hands off each other, but over the years that ship may have sailed. Is it possible to make great sex last—or come back to embrace us again?

You can have a real shot at more fully enjoying your long-term relationship—including enjoying some marvelous sex after 50—but it won't happen automatically. It likely will take some effort you didn't know you'd have to exert and perhaps some new skills you haven't had a chance to learn before. Your payoffs in the second half of life can include more pleasure, love, happiness, friendship, intimacy, and maybe even better sex. Not only that, it may help you be healthier and perhaps even live longer. We'd say that's the bargain of the half-century!

Lover: Lost and Found

QUESTION: *My husband and I started out so much in love; we couldn't get enough of each other. Even after twenty-two years of marriage, we still like spending time together and make love about once a week. I thought when the kids were gone, I'd start enjoying sex more, but to be honest, it's gotten so boring in bed I can't wait to just get it over with. I even make excuses to get out of it. I feel pretty crummy for not liking sex more, but what can I do? My husband would be crushed if he knew.*

—Rosario, 51

If you're bored in bed, you're bored in bed. It's just a fact, not a measure of anyone's self-worth. Boring sex happens in many long-term relationships. In the beginning, hormones give us lust, romantic love, and keep sex exciting. But over time, as we are busy living our complicated lives, our bodies change, we change, and passion tends to slip away. By the time we realize that our connection with our best bed buddy is disappearing, few people know how to get it back.

Even if you still love your partner, that early, whirly "in love" sensation inevitably gets replaced with a complex mix of friendship and annoyance, commitment and disappointment, tenderness and resentment, deep bonding and often just plain boredom. What started out as a quality you loved (for example, your partner's excitement for life or their ability to be thoughtful before taking action), may now have become an irritant (Why is he always so hyperactive? or Why can't she just make up her mind?).

If you haven't had good sex for a while, it's no wonder that you still don't. Sex in a long-term relationship at midlife and beyond doesn't usually get better on its own; *it takes some conscious effort.* You said you still like your husband's company, and that's a big plus. (You'd be surprised how many long-term couples don't like each other.) But even that may eventually slip away unless you learn some new communication skills and perhaps take a few risks. It may seem like your husband's responsibility to fix this problem, but it's really up to you. He probably doesn't even know you are unsatisfied. You can continue down this dull, passionless path or begin a journey toward a sexier, more pleasurable future. This new child-free stage you are in now could be a perfect time to tell him the truth about what you are experiencing, take steps to reconnect, and rekindle some genuine fire in the bedroom. It won't all happen in a weekend, but it certainly can be done—if you are willing to make the effort.

Are you?

Lazy About Loving

No matter how much we each give to our children, jobs, careers, or homes, most of us are just plain lazy about loving our partners. It's not that we are willfully lazy or that we don't dearly love our mates. In fact, many of us would do almost anything to save our lovers' lives, but keeping our relationships in tip-top shape is not high on most people's to-do list. We tend to think that love and sex shouldn't take that much effort (it didn't when we were young), and we often don't have the skills or the role models to learn how to give and get what we really want. Instead, we get complacent, take our relationships for granted, and sex becomes routine. Routines, although comforting, can also be boring.

Back when love was new, no one ever told us that one day it would take work, and even if they did, who would believe it? The truth is that no one is ever fully ready for a long-term relationship. Being *in* a relationship year in, year out is what teaches you *how* to be in one. You don't know what you are getting yourself into until you get there and learn to live through the ups and downs. Over time, people change and not always as you hoped. That wonderful person you committed yourself to so many years ago has disappeared, and so has the you who originally said "I do." Some couples split up, while others leave emotionally even if they stay together physically. If you want love and good sex to last and grow, the two new people who you are today will probably have to make some effort to create your new bonding glue. True intimacy and great sex take effort, and staying in love requires an action plan (and maybe even some sex toys; see Chapter 9).

Dr. Dorree Says:

No long-term relationship would last if one's brain didn't kick in when you wanted to leave and you didn't say to yourself, *Stay and work it out.*

Intimacy and How You Sleep

How and where you sleep in the bed may say something interesting about you, like how much space you need in your relationship and what your boundaries are. Which one of the following describes you?

You Sleep Intertwined with Your Partner All Night

Some partners, especially in comfortable, long-term relationships, sleep close and even turn with their partners unconsciously in their sleep. It's as if, no matter what happens during the day, even if they are at odds, they find comfort in each other's body warmth and connection at night. When sleeping apart, these couples often do just fine alone, but when together (no matter how big the bed) they intertwine and turn together as one. This is no guarantee that their relationship will last any longer than others, but for some it does provide deep comfort and body nurturance during sleep.

You Like to Cuddle or Spoon for a while, Then Sleep Apart

Many people like pre- and post-sleep cuddling for comfort and connection, without sticking together like Velcro all night. They also enjoy pre- and post-sex caressing or spooning (as opposed to "roll-over-and-go-away-after-sex" manners). When they are actually sleeping, however, they prefer their own space.

You Keep a Toe or a Hand Touching or Nearby

This can provide reassurance that all is well, without your feeling confined by the other person. It may also be a compromise sleep style for bed partners who have different needs for comfort and connection—that is, where one wants more and the other wants less. Or maybe you both just like to know you are not alone, yet still sleep apart.

You Stay Mostly on Your Side of the Bed

Even when your partner is gone, you have your special place. This is your territory and your comfort zone. You meet your partner in the middle of the bed for sexual activity—often involving intercourse, which is pretty hard to accomplish long distance—or you both get into a pattern of one partner, usually the sex initiator, coming over to visit the more sexually passive, noninitiator's side. Light sleepers (like many women after menopause) may sleep in their own corners to avoid their partner's movements or noises.

Some couples may even end up sleeping in separate rooms, with occasional "visits" in each other's beds. For some, sleeping together is too physically or emotionally uncomfortable, or both. Or maybe it's just the snoring!

You Sleep in the Center of the Bed

With or without your partner, the center is yours! It's your world and your territory and you like spreading out. You are fortunate if your partner is willing and able to fit around your needs (both physically and emotionally). To make this work in most beds, your partner needs to be relatively smaller than you. If he or she needs more room, you could try putting two beds together. Otherwise, one of you may not get enough rest (or even enough power in the relationship).

Changing Your Sleep Style

Some couples alter their sleep styles (on purpose or unconsciously) due to illness, anger, boredom, or a host of other reasons. But most couples tend to fall into a pattern and stick with it, and it is common for this routine not to suit both partners equally. Given that we spend about a third of our lives in bed, with whom we sleep and how comfortable our style are worth thinking about.

A good example of a sleep style that had to change was Emelia and José's. Brought up devoutly religious, the couple prayed together nightly, clad up to their necks in nightclothes, before each going to sleep on their own side of the bed. Emelia

tossed and turned and eventually
slept; José popped his ear plugs in
and fell asleep listening to his iPod.

It was only later in therapy, while
exploring their sexless marriage, that
this routine slowly changed at Dr.
Dorree's gentle urging. She asked the
partners to consider praying first, then
talking, then taking off a little bit of
clothing, and then going to sleep next
to each other—sans ear plugs. Slowly,
over the course of many months, they
removed more and more clothing
until they wore none. At that point,
they started sexual activity, not out of desire, but as a once-a-week
homework task. Emelia wanted it more than José. With time,
they succeeded.

Postgame analysis, why did this work? For deeply rooted childhood reasons, José was afraid to connect to the woman he loved
dearly. He had to think his way through changing his behavior
first, and then later his emotions could catch up. As with sports,
trial and error and then practice, you can make it work.

I Want My Wife Back!

QUESTION: *I don't understand what happened to my marriage.
I thought it would last forever and now we are miserable and haven't had sex for months. How do I get
my old wife back?*

—JACKSON, 54

Like it or not, not one of us is getting our former wives or husbands back. Among the many things they don't tell you when you're young is the fact that, even if you stay with the same woman or man for your entire life, there is really no such thing as a single long-term relationship. You are actually having a series of many sequential relationships with the same person. Just like our ever-changing bodies, you change, she changes, and your relationship changes. Even if you just became aware of it, your relationship has been changing all along and it will continue to change into the future.

The good news is that you can have a big impact on where your relationship will go next. The first step is facing facts. If you or your partner is dissatisfied, then that is probably a good place to start. Sometimes, the very thing you loved about a partner in the beginning becomes the thing you can't stand about them now. ("He used to finish my sentences, now he doesn't let me speak.") Or the comfort of the relationship allows deeper issues to be exposed.

Here are some of the more common stressors that typically challenge relationships. Try choosing the ones that most impact yours.

- Damaged dreams
- Poor communication
- Emotional, physical, or sexual neglect or abuse
- Infidelity or broken trust that has not been addressed or worked through
- More anger, arguing, bickering, or resentment than fun and joy
- Financial or family worries or differences of opinions about these matters

- Prolonged stress or emotional distress such as depression or anxiety
- Addictions or prolonged use of sleep medication
- Illness
- Boredom
- Unsatisfying sexual connection

Given that none of us are perfect, that we all have our issues, and we each are constantly growing and changing at our own rates (making it hard to even live with *ourselves* sometimes), it is a wonder that long-term relationships survive and thrive at all!

It can be very helpful for each partner to do their personal psychological work, as well as work together as a couple. Some great resources are the books and workshops by Harvel Hendrix for healing childhood issues that may be impinging on your adult relationships, particularly first marriages.

What Color Is Your Partnership?

Take your relationship pulse and check your couple heartbeat by asking yourself which of the following partnership styles best describes you.

Happy Beyond Your Wildest Dreams

You have either just met or you and your partner have learned how to make your relationship truly burn with a bright flame. Sex can be comforting, satisfying, spiritual, or "rockets' red glare." You know how to be intimate with each other and are good friends. If you've been a couple for many years, consider taking your show on the road, or at least mentoring others in your community. All people can learn from what you have to share and what has made your relationship work so well for you. You have maintained and grown love, and that's what makes the world go 'round. Spread your wisdom where you can.

> **Dr. Dorree Says:**
>
> It's hard enough for most people to live with themselves. Double the equation and look at the complexity. Therefore, most relationships bump, slip, and slide between smooth sailing and rough waters—and so does sex.

Life Is Pretty Good

You and your partner have closeness and are respectful of each other. You touch and talk a lot, and sometimes sex can sizzle. Stress can get you down and annoyances may creep in, but mostly life is good. You can keep the good times rolling by sharing meals together, making time for making love, looking for ways to connect and talk. Also find ways to keep your individual interests alive, as well as those you share together. Make time for yourself and each other. Talk about what knots you up. Seek opportunities for positive connections and words of love. Remain present, and aware of ways to help grow and support your relationship.

Walking a Tightrope

You have some pleasure and satisfaction in your relationship, but also some serious annoyances and challenges. The good times usually outweigh the bad. But you can get pretty angry or disappointed, and you either retreat into silence or blow up when you wish you wouldn't. Sex still has its good moments, but not as often as you or your partner would like. Sometimes you're not so sure whether or not you still care. You feel that there is still potential for greater satisfaction and happiness, but that neither of you risk reaching for it. Your dreams have tarnished, but when you are together and relaxed, the dull patina of your connection falls away and you can glow. Sometimes you even laugh together. Keep it and grow it by taking vacations together, going on date nights (and days), and going beyond your usual conversations. The ideas and tips in Chapters 5 and 6 may be all you need to erase some of your troubles and bring more joy into your relationship. Actively look for more reasons to laugh and more time to cuddle.

Hanging In

You don't have much pleasure and often feel dissatisfied. Many days (and nights) seem bleak. Sex is boring or very infrequent. Perhaps your vagina is dry or unresponsive, or your hard-on won't last (even though you have no trouble masturbating). Your eye may be wandering for romance elsewhere. Perhaps you've even had an affair. You don't know how to make your relationship better, yet you don't want to leave. You've got a history and a long-term investment, so you still hold out hope. This is an ideal time to get outside counseling or professional help. You loved your partner once. Perhaps you can get reacquainted and learn the new skills that will have made hanging in through this rough patch worth the effort.

Rock Bottom

You are probably missing the fulfillment of basic relationship needs and may be feeling pain, rage, or intimacy emptiness. Sex is lifeless, if it exists at all. You may be thinking about a trial separation or divorce. You may want to learn why things are this empty for you and whether or not it's worth learning the skills to change it. Will you stay or leave? The help of a close friend, counselor, clergy, or therapist may guide you in figuring it out.

Crazy Time

You've decided to leave, but meanwhile you've stopped sleeping, your eating is a mess, and you aren't sure if you can stay sane for much longer. Sex with your partner has become a distant memory. You might not even remember why you got together in the first place. This is a crazy-feeling time; you may be anxious and/or depressed. Sometimes you wonder how to get through the next hour, much less a day. You may even wonder if life is worth living. It's time to make a move with some careful planning. If possible, get professional help along the way. Maybe getting some mood stabilizers, a massage, acupuncture, or exercise would help. Be careful driving, walk carefully so that you don't trip, and watch out not to bump into walls. Don't scare yourself or stop in midstream. Read Chapter 7 for what might lie ahead.

Guess What? Communication Is *Not* the Key

Yes, you read that correctly! People always say communication is the key to improving your relationship, but clearly, that's not true. We're already *always* communicating. Yelling is communicating, abuse is communicating, the raised eyebrows of countless unsaid criticisms are communicating, unfulfilled sex is communicating, and bickering over who didn't put the top on the peanut butter jar or why the toothpaste was squeezed the wrong way is communicating. And we can probably agree that not too much of any of that is helpful for improving relationships, feeling close, or having great sex.

The real key is *honest, positive communication* that makes your relationship better for both of you so that you feel more understood, appreciated, connected, bonded, trusting, and/or turned-on. However, honest, positive communication does not always mean being nice. It does mean learning how to be truthful about your own needs without purposely being hurtful and actively listening to what your partner has to say without getting wounded every time he or she tells you something you would rather not hear.

Truth and authenticity are never easy to achieve because it takes a fairly good understanding of yourself and the courage to reveal your inner workings to someone else. Everyone wants to feel understood, especially by their lover. But since few of us understand ourselves all of the time, how do we learn to help our partners understand us, no less learn how to better understand them? It is a process that requires practice and possibly help. If this was something you could learn in ten easy steps, everyone would be doing it overnight. The truth is that honest, positive communication takes much skill, awareness, effort, and sometimes also the help of a good counselor or therapist; most new learning takes some guidance.

Twitter Is Not Intimacy

In this age of instant messaging, e-mail, and texting, it's important to remember that you can't tweet your way to a deeper connection with your partner just with quick conversations or short emotional outbursts. Honest, positive, intimacy-building communication is a back-and-forth dialogue between two equally important people with a common goal of creating more mutual understanding. Even if no agreements are immediately reached, each person wants to be heard, not just rebutted. Be respectful and generous in your listening. After you get a chance to say what you think or feel, you can "close the loop" by listening, being thoughtful, and responding. The idea is not simply to say "I hear you," which is where most people stop, but to demonstrate your active listening by mirroring back what has been said and building on it, linking it to yourself, and then passing it back to the other person with something added that moves you both to the next step.

For example, if your partner says, "I'm tired of talking about having sex. When are we going to start actually making love more often?" you can say, "I hear that you want to have sex more often, and I am hoping that eventually I will, too. Right now I don't have the same desire level that you do. I'd like to tell you more about how I think we can change that. Would that be okay, or would you like to talk about something else?" When you close the loop in this way, even if your partner doesn't want to talk about it now, hopefully he or she will feel understood, respected, and not forced into a conversation he or she isn't ready to have. In fact, your partner might even want to keep talking!

Why Can't He Hear Me!?

QUESTION: *I keep trying to tell my husband why I am so unhappy, but all he hears is that I think he is wrong in some way, which causes no end of arguing and gets us nowhere. Everyone says to keep talking about it, but how can I get him to actually listen to me? He manages to hear the football scores just fine.*

—LUCY, 49

We know it's an overused generalization, but the idea that men are from Mars and women are from Venus really does have some merit. Couples often get into communication conflicts without knowing whether they are differing about style or about content. As with sex, many men prefer to cut right to the chase, while women may tend to talk on and on. Most men are fixers and believe they are being helpful when they try to solve a problem, while women tend to talk in order to be understood, not necessarily to have the specific problem solved (in fact, not feeling understood *is* her main problem, not the original issue). So a woman may tend to keep talking (trying to be understood), and a man may just hear that there are more and more problems he is failing to solve (criticisms that cut deep), until tempers flare or resentments build. It's as if a straight line and circle are trying to get together.

There are other reasons for miscommunication. Sometimes one person keeps interrupting the other because he thinks he knows what is about to be said. Or some people, although they don't mean to, either tune out what they don't want to hear or are so busy forming their counter-responses, like trial attorneys, that they never fully hear what their partners are saying.

To stay away from courtroom debate, it can help to have a face-to-face discussion over a relaxed dinner before your hurt overtakes you and even more dissatisfaction develops in your relationship. Honest communication and active listening are difficult and almost always take some practice. An online course, a few sessions with a professional, or reading the tips offered in this chapter or other books can get you started, but it does take practice.

Consciously or unconsciously, people may block or avoid effective communication for any number of reasons, including:

• fear of feeling vulnerable or exposed
• fear of being rejected or abandoned
• lack of positive communication skills (no one teaches you this stuff)
• anxiety about the other person's anger or disapproval
• fear of being discovered as a fraud
• fear of revealing a painful secret (most couples do keep some secrets, small or large, from their partners)
• feeling shame about something they think is bad about themselves
• feeling guilty about something they did

Just one of these unresolved issues can derail an otherwise positive attempt at discussing a relationship issue or proposing solutions. Remember, we are all such tender creatures beneath our skin, some more so than others. Some of us have a "criticism allergy" and break out in aggressive arguing at the mere whiff of it. Others may react to criticism by withdrawing and seething instead of boiling over, later exploding over something seemingly minor. If your partner is sensitive to criticism (many people are), take extra care to protect his or her more fragile areas so you can help each other hear and say what needs to be said. Remember, kindness and generosity go a long way.

Can You Hear Me Now?

Ladies, if you sometimes think your man seems deaf, dumb, and blind, that may actually be partially true, at least the deaf part is pretty common.

Many men as they age tend to lose some of their hearing at the higher range where a woman's voice may mostly reside. If your guy seems to be missing some of what you've been saying lately, there's a good chance he might benefit from a hearing test. Partial hearing loss is far more common than most people realize. Countless arguments and even divorces occur because neither partner realizes that not everything said is being heard. This might be even worse in the comfort of your own home, where a woman may speak at lower decibels, until frustration leads to screaming—either way, she doesn't get heard.

Here's a quick fix: Face each other when you talk. The combination of having a direct line of hearing from lips to ears, as well as the visual information that comes from seeing someone speaking, can add up to much better odds of actually being heard.

And if you need a boost, be open to the possibility of trying a hearing aid. These helpful devices have become remarkably sophisticated and small. As part of the first generation to be raised on rock 'n roll and powered motors, we all face the increased possibility of needing hearing aids, more than our parents. Did you know that former Boomer president Bill Clinton wears one in each ear?

Building Your Communication Toolbox

Honest and effective communication takes tools, skills, and practice. Here are some ways to let the things you say nurture and grow your relationship.

Use "I" statements. Take ownership of your feelings and thoughts. State your personal beliefs and feelings clearly and plainly. For example, instead of "You are so loud and annoying. Why do you keep bothering me?" you can say "I felt scared when you slammed the door. I would really like it if you could please be gentler when you leave." (Follow the phrase "I feel" with an actual feeling word, like sad, mad, bad, glad, and other feeling words, not a criticism, such as "I feel you are really stupid.")

Avoid blame. Stick with what happened and how it affected you, not what a mess you think the other person is. Avoid saying "you always" or "you never." Besides being blaming, it's also probably inaccurate.

Be positive and focus on what you want. "I love it when you touch my shoulder when you walk past me." Or use a "you" compliment: "Your smile makes me happy." Turn a negative into a positive. Instead of saying "I hate it when you're late," try "I really like it when you pick me up on time. It makes me feel loved."

Be direct. "Would you please give me a shoulder rub? I feel so much better when it's your special touch."

Reveal yourself. "I get a tingling feeling when you are near me." Or "I have a secret. I used to get sick when I smelled hot dogs cooking. I still don't do so well even when you cook them at home. I always felt uncomfortable telling you why I want to walk out." (Self-revelation doesn't have to start with big things.)

Be honest and offer positive solutions. "I have never liked your giving me oral sex and I've always been afraid to hurt your feelings. But if we try starting on my thighs, I might be able to learn." Or "I think that shade of green is not the best for you. Let's see what color shirt will show off your handsome face."

Be patient and kind. "Thank you for trying to be gentler in bed. I know how hard it is to change."

When Intimacy Is Missing

QUESTION: *I think I know what intimacy is, or at least I know what it isn't. My partner, Willa, keeps telling me how happy she is in our relationship. We have a great time and tons of fun when we're doing stuff together, like going dancing or strolling through a park. But there's a closeness missing for me that isn't missing for her. We've been together thirty-three years and I love my partner. I don't want to hurt her. I've read more "how to" books than I can count, and Willa has even read a few that I've left on her side of the bed. What is missing? What can I do about it?*

—MARINA, 63

Are you lonely? Do you have enough of your own interests to fulfill you? Are you expecting too much from your partner? Or is intimacy, which comes from self-revelation and ongoing trust, really missing? If so, you can try some of the communication tips and ideas offered in this chapter. It is difficult to feel close to another person without taking risks to reveal yourself and give your life partner a chance to really know you and accept you. Have you been so careful about not hurting your partner that perhaps you have not been as open about your inner self as you might be? There is nothing quite like letting your partner see all sides of you (and loving you anyway) to make you both feel closer than ever.

Emotional Intimacy

Everyone wants to feel respected, worthy, whole, and accepted. Couples feel the most secure when their closest relationships feel comfortable and safe. Each partner wants to feel accepted and not judged. Sometimes, fear of losing one's partner or fear of upsetting them (which might lead to losing them), can hold people back from fully revealing themselves. By not expressing their feelings, they believe they can avoid the pain of loss, or at least limit the pain. But by not being your total self, you are already losing something, and either way loss hurts.

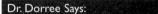

Dr. Dorree Says:

Intimacy can be elusive. Like good theater or soul-stirring jazz, you just know it when you feel it.

And in the meantime, what you've really lost is the everyday pleasure that true love and emotional intimacy can bring. Living in fear of future loss stops you from enjoying the present.

Connection and closeness nurture couples. The sense of safety and care promotes stable and growing relationships. At midlife, you have the time you may not have had earlier in your life to get in touch with and share your emotions with your partner. Sharing feelings, hopes, dreams, fears, and needs builds emotional intimacy. One reason you are in a relationship is to feel valued and loved. You also want to know that your significant other is emotionally available.

How can partners build emotional intimacy? There are no simple answers and each relationship is unique. Here are some basic elements that emotionally intimate couples tend to share.

- **Open communication** of feelings and facts.
- **Trust.** Opening up is easier in an atmosphere of trust. Trust comes from care, compassion, empathy, consideration, kindness, and acceptance—both of the other person and yourself. Self-acceptance allows you to bring a whole, intact person to the relationship that you want to have.
- **Self-acceptance.** Self-acceptance does not mean adhering to some perfect image. It means loving who you are— flaws, strengths—and all that makes you uniquely who you are. Almost no one knows how to feel that secure, so self-acceptance is an ongoing project. We all have secret insecurities; sometimes they are even secret from ourselves.
- **Quality time.** Quality time together creates couplehood. Intimacy doesn't develop if you experience only a few minutes of together time. Schedule quality time so you can share significant moments in and out of bed with your partner. It takes effort, awareness, commitment, and time. And yes, you can make the time.
- **Put your relationship first.** Put your couple first by following the "inverted pyramid" (described later in the chapter). You may be surprised how much easier everything becomes.

Spiritual Intimacy

Lovers and poets have written about this illusive experience for as long as there have been words. Spiritual intimacy underlies all other intimacy, emotional and physical. Spiritual intimacy is not the same as being religious. Think of it as the union of separates, a deep and personal connection with the universe, the earth, mind/body, self, your partner, and others. When you accept yourself and experience spiritual intimacy, you may be physically alone, but you don't feel lonely.

Finding ways to create spiritual intimacy or spiritual solace are challenging for most of us. It may require carving out quiet time (and perhaps practicing a discipline). It may include intercessory prayer (talking to a divine presence) or contemplative prayer (which is practiced in many ancient traditions and is like meditation). Other ways of slowing down and opening oneself to the possibilities of spiritual connection include tai chi, qigong, types of yoga that focus on breathing or body flow (as opposed to the more competitive sports like boxing), time immersed in nature, mindfulness practices taught in many schools and spiritual centers, biofeedback, and breathing-based exercises—anything that helps bring you peace and a feeling of closeness with something beyond yourself. Addictions, such as alcoholism or cigarette smoking, may decrease anxiety but are not a positive way to meet your spiritual and emotional needs.

Intimacy Takes Courage

Taking steps toward more intimacy with your partner can be intimidating, even frightening for some people. It was for Skip and Ann. They always had a very passionate love life together. But passion isn't always a predictor of pleasure. Skip and Ann fought frequently and used passionate sex to assuage their anger and even to make up. Both had orgasms that were physically satisfying, but their hearts grew increasingly empty and there was a considerable edge to their daily interactions.

A lifetime of this pattern of angry, empty sex had left them afraid of being emotionally vulnerable or fully honest with each other. Now the couple is in their mid-60s, and without hormone-driven sex to hold their relationship together, they have become lost and disconnected from each other.

A friend suggested that they see a counselor, which they finally agreed to do. But their road to intimacy was not easy. Emotional disrobing in front of each another can be far more frightening than physically getting undressed. Long-held fears or secrets, words not said, or smoldering resentments take their toll. New intimacy requires new honesty. It takes courage to become vulnerable, risk rejection, speak your truth, and learn to touch in new ways.

Your Partner Is Not Psychic

Take responsibility for what you want and find out how your partner wants to be treated. Make an effort to be more sensual with each other. Show your partner what you want in bed. Touch, touch, touch! The skin is the largest sex organ and is often overlooked. Try different ways of touching each other all over the body. Perhaps experiment with various safe items and sensations, like a feather, a silk scarf, an ice cube, flower petals, maybe even whipped cream! Play dressup if that excites you, or just wear something fun and comfortable, it's all good if it makes you both feel good.

In this age of technology, we have the tools and toys to make sex easier, more fun, and even possible for some people (see Chapter 9). And remember, fantasy—either as your own private thoughts, shared with your partner in bed, or even acted out during sex—is a great sex energizer for both men and women.

Why Is Finding Intimacy So Difficult?

QUESTION: *I keep trying to quiet myself but it just doesn't work. Besides, I love living with a live-wire, whirlwind who never slows down.*

—RANI, 51

Many of us are simply not well-trained to meet emotional needs—our own or those of the people we love. If you haven't been exposed to it and haven't regularly seen it in action before, how would you know how to do it? Where would you have learned?

Your parents, or whoever raised you, were your primary role models. Were they intimate? Presumably, while you were growing up, you didn't live in their bedroom, but how did they behave outside the bedroom? Did they reflect the ingrained messages from our culture that don't support intimacy, or those from a previous era when intimacy was not considered as essential and relationships were based mostly on functional roles?

If so, you are a pioneer forging new ground. Life does not come with a how-to intimacy manual. It takes life learning to acquire new skills. Consider some of the following suggestions.

- Acknowledge, express, and discuss feelings—your own and your partner's.
- Feel and express love through words, deeds, touch, sex (with or without penetration or orgasm).
- Stick with a hard conversation or tough topic, stay in the room, and be appropriately humorous or serious when words touch you.
- Be sensitive and accepting of your emotions and those of others. Even though we live in a world of let everything

hang out reality shows, society at large still sends messages that say: don't cry in public, tough it out, emotions are for wimps, expressing feelings is a sign of weakness, and other messages that tell us not to feel anything.

Learning to open up and connect takes time. Your partner isn't the same person as you and has needs that may be quite different from yours. (If you are in a long-term relationship, you already know that in spades.) Learning to understand your partner's way of thinking and responding, and how they react to the world in emotional terms, may take patience, openness, and new skills.

Remember, marriage is always a work in progress—the good ones, that is. The bad ones don't work and don't progress.

Fair Fighting Is Fine (As Long As You Make Up)

Mean, dirty, or unfair fighting, or fighting just for the sake of fighting, are not intimacy builders, even if you have post-fight make-up sex at the end. On the other hand, expressing dissatisfactions in appropriate ways, even if it involves loud and emotional conversations, can free energy for love to flourish. A fight that ends with greater understanding, an agreement for change, or even just a promise to continue the discussion at another time is a productive fight even if it is unpleasant at the time.

Dr. Dorree Says:

Intimacy isn't always genteel and quiet. Sometimes intimacy and love include arguing, zealous conversation, touching, dancing, crying, singing, passionate sex, and slow, tender sex. It's all intimacy if you share a deep connection together.

Think of your relationship like a resilient but also potentially vulnerable child. Studies show that children who grow up in tumultuous homes usually do well in life if fighting is tempered by love or they see adults make up after disagreements. (Think of the stereotypical Mediterranean home filled with expressive, even explosive emotion and great love.) On the other hand, kids who come from families that rarely express emotion or who see only arguing that does not end with reconciliation don't do as well. The ability to actively "kiss and make up" seems to be the difference.

Long-term relationships always have some friction. The trick is to rub each other the wrong way on occasion and still be able to bond together and be sensual, loving, and sexual the majority of the time. Remember, *foreplay begins in the morning* (see Chapter 5). Everything you say and do together either adds or subtracts from the connection and sex you may have later. Think about what kind of foreplay you are creating each day. When you fight, make up! Sometimes love *does* mean saying I'm sorry.

Is Arguing Good for Us? Let's Not Fight About It!

After studying 192 married couples over a period of seventeen years, researchers at the University of Michigan found that the spouses who expressed anger lived longer than those who bottled it up. Other research, however, suggests that resolving conflicts without any arguing at all is better for your health.

The British comedy group Monty Python begs to differ. Here's a paraphrasing of a small section of their hilarious sketch called "The Argument Clinic."

A man comes into the Argument Clinic, announcing, "I've come here for a good argument." The attendant answers, "No, you didn't. You just came here for a regular argument; you have no interest in a good one."

Perhaps the most complex aspect of keeping a loving relationship alive is learning how to be two separate, growing individuals and still come together as a team. People are ever-changing, life is not static, and no matter how perfectly you may plan, life always eventually throws you a curveball. A loving couple can learn how to catch curveballs and even how to grow the game.

Man: "No, please don't just contradict me. An argument is not merely a contradiction."

Attendant: "It can be."

Man: "No, it can't. An argument is a series of statements to establish a proposition."

Attendant: "No, it isn't."

Man: "Yes, it is! It's not just contradiction!"

Attendant: "Look, if I argue with you, I must take up a contrary position."

Man: "True, but that's not just saying, 'No, it isn't.'"

Attendant: "Yes, it is."

Man: "No, it isn't!" (short pause) *"Damn it!"*

Does Your Relationship Pass the Personal Pleasure Test?

Barry has been living with Bill for four years. The two lovers get along well in their shared business, a high-end retail store that they co-own. They don't fight much at home and live what might seem like an idyllic life, full of friends, sophisticated cultural outings, and social events. The trouble is Barry is not happy in the bedroom, beautifully appointed as it may be. Bill tends to be mechanical and routine, at least through Barry's eyes, and the passion is gone. They have every ingredient for a wonderful life, except for the one thing that Barry wants most: intimacy.

What's the one thing you want most? Are you getting it? When you experience pleasure with your partner, do you feel love, trust, respect, and satisfaction? When these feelings are not there, even if the sex is technically flawless, we tend to feel pain, disappointment, unhappiness, and the loss of love. This is no minor consideration, especially after 50. One of the big shifts in the second half of life is that desires, feelings, and thoughts take on equal, if not greater roles than our hormones. So pay attention to the quality of your interactions. They may be telling you something important. Dissatisfaction doesn't necessarily mean your relationship is over, but it may need your attention, effort, and even some bravery in order to improve and flourish.

The Nose Knows

If you are confused about whether or not you can still be physically attracted to your partner even if your relationship were to improve, here's a quick check that is surprisingly accurate. A study of people participating in couple's therapy to solve marital problems found that participants who reported liking their partners scent at the start of therapy were significantly more likely than other couples to stay together, even though both groups had months of therapy and other relationship support. Apparently, the power of smell to attract or repel is a better predictor of future desire than many of us may realize.

How to Talk About Sex

QUESTION: *Everyone always says to talk about what you want, but they never tell you how! I either keep it all to myself, or if I do bring up something that is bothering me in bed, it only starts an argument. What's so good about that?*

—SANDY, 60

Talking about sex can be a delicate, even challenging task for most people, and if you have any added issues, such as fears, illnesses, or unresolved relationship problems, it might feel twice as hard for you. Here are some tips for talking more effectively about sex:

- Always, always, always talk about sex issues and other problems *away* from the bedroom or wherever you usually make love. Set aside a relaxed time when neither of you are too tired. If you think the conversation may get heated, try meeting in a private location in a public place (it's easier to keep your cool in a restaurant than in your bathrobe). Don't expect to necessarily resolve everything in one conversation. There's no rush.
- When speaking, avoid criticism or blame. Remember to use "I" statements and to focus on your feelings and thoughts, not on evaluating your partner. For example, "I feel lonely when you roll over and go right to sleep after intercourse."
- Encourage your partner to open up and really listen to what you both are saying. The goal is not just to get what you want but to find what will work for both of you. Ask him or her for ideas and offer some of your own. It takes honesty and courage to gently negotiate a new way of being sexual together. Be kind and loving. Assure your

partner that he or she is still attractive and loved. We all need that at every age.

- If you find talking too difficult, you can try communicating what you want nonverbally. The next time you're having sex, use your hands to guide your partner in what you want. This won't solve most relationship problems, but it can teach your partner new ways to please you and even a small change can begin the process of feeling closer, perhaps making it easier to talk in the future.

Who Will Make the First Move?

QUESTION: *Why do I have to be the one to fix this? He is the one who is ignoring my needs, so why do I have to do all the work? This would be so much easier with a different partner!*

—EMILY, 52

Whose needs aren't getting met, yours or his? The one who is the least satisfied is the one who has the most reason to do something about it (unfair, we know, but true). But making the first move is not equivalent to doing all the work; it's just taking responsibility for breaking the logjam and getting things rolling. Long-term couples often find themselves in a stalemate: "Why should I do anything if you're not doing anything?" Maybe you have years of resentment or a habit of fighting. Maybe both partners feel wronged by some past indiscretions and now neither party wants to give an inch. But relationships are not financial transactions in which everything has to equal out in order to reconcile the books. If something isn't working and you want it to be better, there comes a time to put the past behind you and see what you can create in the here and now.

Women often want to improve the relationship, and they can begin the change process and educate their partners (gently and with respect). Men want to be happy, too, and they can learn with information and education. It doesn't matter who starts the process as long as you both end up happier together. Begin by talking and continue communicating regularly to build your skills. What has happened that has made you so angry, disappointed, or hurt? Are you giving your relationship the time and energy it needs to flourish, or are you coming home at the end of the day, both exhausted and needy, having given your all at the office or to the kids, and only have leftovers for each other? Or maybe he simply doesn't know what you like in bed, or she doesn't realize that something she keeps saying is hurtful.

Whatever the issue, even a tiny change can be transformational. Sometimes you need the help of a therapist, but not always. Work at it and change your habits. So many people get depressed and want to quit, instead of using this time to rebuild, renegotiate, and reconnect. Mountains of research confirms that, in general, couples who stay together despite the ups and downs of life are happier, healthier, and have more frequent sex than people who split up.

The bottom line is that marriage is good for you. If you possibly can stay together, try to find a way. So what if you have to make the first move forward? Do you really think moving out will be so much easier? Either way, it all takes effort. You might as well see what you can do before you quit.

Renegotiate Your Relationship

If there's one thing you can count on in this whirling world of ours is that all things change. Just since you started reading this book, *you* have changed, both physically and mentally. The idea that your partnership won't change is not only silly, it can hurt you. Committing to a long-term relationship is not like stepping inside a Hallmark card and then spending the rest of your days together trying to stay there, frozen in time. Maintaining a healthy, satisfying, and ever-changing partnership requires conscious renegotiation at each stage.

You can think of the process of renegotiating your relationship like dating again—only with a shared history and the same person. Well, not exactly the same person. You have both morphed into different people from who you were when you met. It's time to get acquainted.

You can set aside some alone time in a pleasant place and begin to talk about how you feel and what you want. Be sure to ask about and listen to what your partner would like, as well. It's not the Me Show, it's the We Show. Keep the conversation as upbeat and positive as possible. It's not especially effective to start your renegotiating process with a list of grievances and complaints. It's better to bring to the

Dr. Dorree Says:

As a practicing therapist for more than three decades, who has also been married, divorced, remarried, a working mom, and a grandmother, and who has listened to tales of woe and wonder, I can tell you from both personal and professional experience that both staying together and not staying together take a lot of effort. If at all possible, staying together in a good relationship is better than splitting up. People are built for togetherness.

table some clarity about what you like and want, not what you dislike. If your partner isn't immediately on board, give him or her reasons why what you are asking for will be good not just for you but for both of you. Paint a positive picture of what you want and "sell it" to your partner in terms he or she can understand and appreciate. This isn't just about getting what you want and need, but also what will be a win-win for both of you.

For example, if you want more date nights and your partner wants more golf, instead of getting into an argument over "what's more important, me or the tee?" how about linking the two together? Find a new golf course you'd like to try and arrange for a special dinner out afterward. The non-golfing partner can shop, read, or get a massage.

Be creative and flexible, but make sure you get what you need and want to feel satisfied with your current relationship. If something isn't working for you, speak up and change it. Let go of the past and be realistic about the future so you can enjoy today with all your heart. That may sound corny, but if the two of you won't put some effort into creating the life and relationship you want, who will?

Dr. Dorree's Motto: "Life Is Too Hard to Do Alone—Reach Out!"

With three-quarters of the U.S. population moving every five years, few of us live close to our extended families or long-term friends. Unless you actively seek out community for fun and support, you may find your relationship bobbing around like a rowboat in an ocean of demands, with only the two of you available for all of life's tasks, from child rearing, financial planning, and household management, to educator, best friend, and confidant. There is so much pressure on the average American couple today, it's quite remarkable that as many people spend their bonus years together as they do

The changes required to make a good relationship even better are difficult to do without outside support. Consider becoming active in a volunteer group, your community, house of worship if you have one, or any place where you can get involved, feel valued, and develop supportive friendships.

If trouble brews, there's no shame in seeking professional help. Turn off your reality TV show and tune in to your own reality. When seeking a good therapist, consider the same suggestions offered in Chapter 5 for finding a good sex therapist. Be the one who makes the call and gets things rolling. Few people realize that it's often the healthiest member of a couple who seeks help first. After all, he or she is willing to admit something's not right. Once in therapy, the other partner will likely need to work at it harder or longer than the one who initiated the help. It all evens out in the end.

Choose someone with good credentials who comes well-recommended and with whom you can comfortably talk. What good is asking for help if you don't trust the person you are telling your secrets to? Most people take more time shopping for a new pair of jeans than finding the right fit when it involves their life and love. Be kind to yourself and put in the effort. It can make all the difference for the rest of your life. And if your partner refuses to go with you—no matter! Simply begin yourself. It only takes one person to change a dance step or develop a new tune.

Friendship Is an Aphrodisiac

QUESTION: *My longtime girlfriend of seventeen years is the love of my life, but we don't make love as much as I'd like, and we're so busy, we just don't have much fun anymore. Maybe people shouldn't stay together this long?*

—DAVID, 56

Moving on to someone new is always an option, but if your partner is really the love of your life, how about sticking around and making it fun again? Being busy with so many tasks and goals, couples often become good co-managers but lose sight of being good friends. If you want your lover back, it will probably take rebuilding your friendship and having some genuine fun together. Studies show that partners in midlife and beyond who share more of their lives outside the bedroom maintain greater intimacy inside the bedroom. So anything you can do to stay active, share interests, and have fun together as a couple can help turn up the heat of your sexual energies, whether it's a weekly date night, a shared hobby, a weekend away once in a while, or a vacation together.

Traveling together can be a great way to connect. It needn't be an expensive trip to Rio de Janeiro. Just a one-night stay away can reap big rewards. If you're a camper, grab your tent. If you're a hiker, grab your walking stick—and maybe your blanket, too, in case you need a cuddling break. Whatever is fun and fits your lifestyle will help build and reinforce the bonds between you.

Even if you've been together for years, you can decide to start dating each other as if you are courting again. Don't just go through the motions, put some effort into it! You can even set a date for sex and then enjoy the building anticipation.

Laugh Yourselves Sexy

Laughter can also be a great aphrodisiac and a wonderful antidote to what ails you. Snuggle up together with a funny movie at home, read joke books out loud to each other, or get creative, like Baxter and Nakieta did. Married for seven years and starting to hit the boredom wall in the bedroom, the couple decided to spend a weekend at a bed-and-breakfast near the beach. Just as they were about to make love, they heard a rhythmic thumping against the thin wall that separated their room from the couple next door. At first, they were unsure what was going on, but when the moaning started it became clear that they weren't the only lovebirds in a new nest for the night. They listened as the passionate banging and moaning grew louder and louder, until Nakieta and Baxter could no longer hold back their giggles from the guilty pleasure of unintentionally eavesdropping on someone else's lovemaking.

They tried to be as quiet as they could, but when moments later the man behind the wall suddenly started snoring as loud as a freight train, they burst into gales of uncontrollable laughter. Like two teenagers who had just sneaked out of the house, the couple made passionate love to each other (careful to pull their bed's headboard away from the wall). Sometimes a thin wall can tear down a boredom wall.

No Time for Love? Build an Inverted Pyramid!

Have you lost your sexy relationship because your lover and yourself are no longer your first (or even your ninth) priority? Have the pushes and pulls of raising kids, running after a career, feeding your family, paying the bills, mowing the lawn, and all the rest of life's demands put you and your partner at the bottom of the heap?

Here's an idea that reverses the way most of us live. (Think about it more than once—it's easy to conceptualize, but not so easy to implement.) Arrange your priorities in an *Inverted Pyramid.* At the base of the pyramid (the pointy end because it is upside down) are you and your mate; next comes your children and family; then your work, social causes, and all the rest. You still have to give at the office, attend the PTA meeting, clean the house, or volunteer in your community, but instead of having nothing but leftovers at home and putting your relationship last, you and your partner are first. Your relationship becomes the foundation, the support, and the source of energy for everything else.

The Make-Time-for-Sex Pyramid

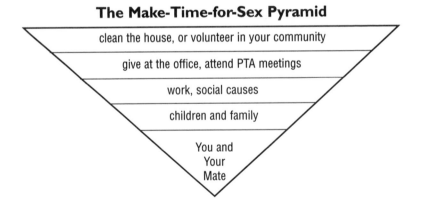

Plan and keep date nights sacred, even if you have to cut back elsewhere. Be creative about how you will spend time together, maybe adding a surprise dress-up lunch out or a romantic weekend rendezvous, so you can remember what your partner looks like out of sweat pants or pajamas. You can't restart a fire without matches or kindling. Take the time to find new ways to make sparks. No one else is going to do it for you. A hot and sexy relationship takes some hot and sexy attention. Like going to a hotel's new bed every once in a while to get away from the often boring bed at home, or trying out some new sex toys or erotica (see Chapter 9).

Getting the Sex You Want

QUESTION: *I'm doing everything I can to make my relationship a priority and make my wife feel like a queen, but it's not having much impact in bed. Where's that hot sex I was hoping for?*

—MONTEL, 52

Sometimes the difference between what you have and what you want is not as far away as you may think. If you are communicating well and your relationship is basically good, but sex is dull, unsatisfying, or too infrequent, even small changes—like those below—can bring improvement.

- Go to bed at the same time. It's hard to make love when one of you is in another room, reading, or watching TV.
- Give gifts of love and appreciation: an unexpected cup of tea, a bottle of wine, flowers for no particular occasion, or a love note (not a toaster because you like toast.) If you don't know what your lover likes, find out! Asking is not "unromantic."
- Add some spice to sex with erotic stories, shared fantasies, pornography, or whatever turns on you (and your partner). If you don't know what you like, experiment and find out.
- Remember that foreplay starts in the morning and lasts all day. Aim to be the lover you'd like to be with the person you love the most.

Make Your Bedroom a Sex Palace

QUESTION: *My wife spends hours every day cleaning the house and yelling at me and the kids to pick up after ourselves. Then we go to sleep at night in a cluttered bedroom full of unfinished projects, give-away bags, out of season stuff, and whatever else lands in there. How can I explain to her that it's hard to feel sexy in a storage bin?*
—DANIEL, 52

Dr. Dorree Says:

When beset by competing demands, remember to take care of yourself and your couplehood first. The two of you are the base from which all else operates. Then come children, family, friends, work, and everything else.

Making the bedroom an inviting and sexy environment when you're busy with kids and careers can be difficult. If you (or your partner) are putting most of your efforts into keeping the rest of the house tidy, the master bedroom can become a catchall, who-cares space where you simply collapse at the end of the day with little energy for anything else. Even many "neat freaks" who keep their homes spotless may have sterile bedrooms that have become sexual deserts.

After the kids move out, or at the start of a new relationship, people at and after midlife have a new opportunity to rethink what their special bed and bedroom can mean for themselves and their intimates. A couple's bedroom can become a sanctuary for comfort, restful sleep, and especially making love. Or it can stay a gloomy, neglected space where rest doesn't come easily—and neither do you! Think carefully about your bedroom and how you use it.

Here are some ideas for making the bed sexy again (or perhaps for the first time).

Create Sexy Atmospherics

Dr. Dorree Says:

There is a difference between what is often the devil-may-care sex of youth and mature lovemaking, which allows more space for consideration, care, and concern.

With money or without, with a whole room makeover or just a new pillowcase, you can begin to create a bedroom that is pleasing to you and your partner, a place of comfort and ease. Add beauty and art if that makes you happy, or leave it wide-open and vacant if that feels more relaxing and calm. Good window coverings shut out the light. If your room is not already quiet, carpeting or even wall hangings can help. If you read in bed, have a good light.

If you're over 50 and single, creating a bedroom for personal comfort can recharge your energy. If you're in a new relationship, you may want to try a fresh decorating scheme that banishes the old cobwebs. And if you're in a long-term relationship, a new start in the bedroom can jump-start your sexual partnership. It can say, "Our relationship is worth making our private space together wonderful."

Sometimes as people get older, bedrooms can start to resemble hospital rooms. Folks set out their glasses, sometimes their teeth, their creams, their pills, perhaps their sexual aids, and other paraphernalia that gets added with added years. Give some thought to how you want to display all this stuff. It helps to have a place for everything. And to make it sexy, it's particularly helpful to keep your sexual aids handy, while stashing your medical aids out of sight. That way the visual message says your bedroom is for sleeping, sex, intimacy, and fun (not a minor medical clinic).

A TV in the bedroom can become competition for love-making. You don't have to ban television entirely (although some people find that helps), but do think about how you use radio, television, and music. Are they a battleground between you and your partner or a shared experience? Does one of you feel left out or rejected? Many people seem to fall in love with their remotes instead of their partners. There's even some scientific evidence that TV rays impact your brain and sleep patterns. Television can be fun, but it's not always a relationship's best friend. Keep your bedroom as private as possible. If you have guests or other family members living at home, your bed and bedroom is the last place to offer them, no matter how generous you may want to be.

Make Your Bed a Passion Playground

Given that you spend up to one-third or more of your life in bed, both sleeping and making love, your bed might be the most important item in your home. If you want your love life to improve, put your money and creativity where your bed is. Today, the bed choices are nearly endless: pillow-top mattress, latex, airbed, memory foam, waterbed, extra-long bed, even beds that have different firmness for each partner. Try various mattresses in the stores or take advantage of a bed that offers an in-home trial. If you can't swing an expensive new bed, make the mattress you have the best it can be, perhaps by adding an inexpensive foam mattress topper for added comfort.

Dress your bed for luxurious comfort. Pillows, comforters, and all the things that many of us didn't have time to think about when we were under 50 can now be a gift to ourselves in the second half of life. If you can afford it, spring for ultrasmooth high-thread-count sheets and high-end, comfortable bedding to pamper yourself in bed. Or shop the clearance tables at department stores, or check out thrift stores for new-to-you sheets and bedding. Even a new pillowcase can change how you feel when you head to bed.

You don't have to give up your flannel nightgown or sleep naked if you don't want to, but do sleep in clothes that are comfortable, easy to remove (in case you get lucky), and are different from what you wore during the day.

Sometimes a small change can have a big impact, as it did for Anita and Bill, both in their 70s. With Anita's bad back and Bill's arthritis in his knees, it had been a long time since the couple had sex. They had tried different positions for intercourse but everything hurt at least one of them. Then Bill, a former engineer, had an idea. He raised the bed to just the right height so that he could stand near the edge of the mattress and not have to lean on his sore knees to make love. And Anita could lay back, legs spread, and enjoy sex without the weight of her husband on top of her during intercourse. Changing the bed changed their sex life. (See sexual position on page 140, standing intercourse.)

You can try this, too, simply by putting inexpensive bed lifters under each corner of your bed to raise the height. They may also make it easier to get in and out of bed.

Create a Sexier Bedtime Routine

QUESTION: *I couldn't stand my husband's terrible snoring another minute so I've been sleeping in the guest room. I love the peace and quiet, but now we rarely see each other. How can we keep the romance alive?*

—BETTY, 57

An estimated 20 percent of American couples do not sleep in the same bed. This is not necessarily a sign of a poor relationship. With age, people are willing to experiment and create their own comfort zones. Some people find that they need more alone time or that their partners' snoring or rolling around in bed really troubles them. There is a difference between sleeping apart because you just don't like each other anymore, and choosing to sleep separately for comfort's sake. If it's the latter, it's important to make the time and effort to meet, greet, and connect with each other for sharing, intimacy, and lovemaking. Even when you sleep in the same bed, if you go to bed at very different times, it helps to make a conscious effort to bond with each other for the sake of your relationship and sex lives. Find some time each day to cuddle and connect in bed, with or without sex.

One way of keeping passion and sex alive is to consider making love in new places, like a night in a hotel, or for those who are adventurous, remembering the passion of your youth on the living room floor, or in front of a fireplace, or maybe even on a kitchen table. If a new environment is a turn-on for you, be creative and find new places to keep sex alive.

Leave Stress at the Door

If you can only do one thing to make your bedroom an oasis for you and your partner, *keep stress out*. If you possibly can, put computers and work papers someplace else, and above all, save all stress-producing conversations (about money, children, sick parents, grandparents, illnesses, and whatever might raise your blood pressure) for outside the bedroom. Once you enter your special space, try to protect yourself and your partner from all sex-chilling stress of any kind.

Be a Lifetime Learner

Learning about love, sex, yourself, and your partner never ends; it's a continuing education. Most of us have been so busy for most of our adult lives with family, work, and all the things it takes to live in the world. So of course we missed a lot of learning time and have some "classes" to make up. It's never too late to learn how to have the best relationship and sex possible. Fairy tales are for kids. Happily ever after only happens with *learning ever after*.

SEVEN

DATING AFTER FIFTY
Plenty of Fish in the Sea

Wouldn't you love somebody to love? The late, great rocker Janis Joplin certainly thought so.

In today's fast-paced, ever-changing world, many people in their 50s, 60s, 70s (and beyond) suddenly find themselves unwillingly and often unexpectedly alone. Unless you want to give up shared sex entirely and live by yourself, the time may come when you are once again (or perhaps for the first time) seeking a partner. At any age, the thought of dating can be both a thrilling and a chilling prospect. Dating after 50 can be a strange, even scary experience, as well as an exciting and empowering adventure.

So much depends on one's attitude, self-confidence, and practical knowledge about how to navigate the after-50 dating world. You ask yourself, am I too old? Where do I look? Is there really anyone for me out there? Will he/she really like me? Am I attractive enough? What will I do? What will I wear? Is it really worth the bother?

And what about sex? If you go out, do you have to put out? Does a man over 50 have different needs from a woman who has lived half a century or more? Do folks after 50 still seek the same things in a partner that they wanted in high school or their last marriages? Do you even know what your needs and desires are?

Most of us don't know exactly what we want. That's why it's called the "dating *game*," as much as that term may make you cringe. The game of dating after 50 is often as much about discovering who *you* are now, at this stage of your life, as it is about finding a good partner. So if you'd rather have a root canal than even think about dating, the first step in the dating game is to understand that *you really can do this.* Even you, "at your age," can learn about yourself and be open to the possibility of finding love and happiness. Whether you are straight, gay, lesbian, bisexual, transgender, or exploring, and no matter how you look, where you live, or what your health status, there are gazillions of single people in the world and many of them could easily be a good match for you. But it doesn't happen automatically. You can't just sit home and expect Mr. or Ms. Right to magically appear at your door. There are plenty of fish in the sea, but you do have to leave the office or your house to find them. Dating after 50 takes some research, smart thinking, a cautiously open heart, and the willingness to learn more about yourself on route to your future.

Dating Is Like Job Hunting

Bear with us if this sounds less than romantic, perhaps even too pragmatic, but finding your match is sort of like job hunting, only more complicated. Like a job search, you might get lucky the first time out, or you may have to invest some significant time and effort into sorting through the possibilities. As with job hunting, it helps to know yourself and your goals, and be persistent. And just as with the often tedious task of looking for a job, if finding the right partner starts taking a lot longer than you hoped, you can always take a little break from your search (a vacation) before starting your hunt again. It's possible that with fresh eyes and more dating experience, you might want to change your resume (what you are presenting to the world) or even the kind of person you are searching for. Dating, like job hunting, evolves based on what you learn as you go.

But unlike job hunting, looking for a potential mate involves more of you than just what you want to show the world about yourself. When you begin to date, especially if you are looking for a lasting love affair with a potential life partner, *all of you* is on the line—body, mind, and heart. This is the part that makes dating seem so scary that you may want to turn back before you even begin. Dating takes courage! Luckily, at your age, you probably have more courage than you realize. Just think of all you have been through. Dating could be the next great chapter in your unfolding life story. This can be your time to turn the page and see what happens next!

Fear Factor

QUESTION: *Do I really want to start dating again at this stage of life? It takes so much work to find someone new and then put in all that time and effort to see if they're really the right person. It's all so exhausting and I've*

*had so many hurts. I'm starting to wonder if it is it
really worth the bother.*

—LISA, 63

Faced with dating again after 50, you might want to just
pull the covers over your head and sleep alone forevermore.
That fine, if it's what you really want. But are you sure you are
not just scared? Many mature women and men remember dating in their earlier years, and let's just say their recollections are
not entirely filled with glee. The same things that made dating so nerve-racking when we were younger can feel twice as
terrifying now. No one wants to get hurt, or worse, get hurt
once more. Whether you've been widowed, divorced, in a
long-term relationship that ended, or in a series of short-lived
affairs that didn't last, just about every after-50 dater remem-
bers enough prior heartbreak to make a grown elephant cry.

But leaving your past behind and inventing your own future
is the irresistible lure of dating. Instead of staying in a box of
bad memories, you are giving yourself the chance to blaze new
trails. Yes, the unknown can be frightening, but unless you
want to stay stuck in the same old rut, you may as well forge
ahead. What do you have to lose? Even if things don't go
exactly as you'd like, it is all part of the "free" education here
on planet earth that continues throughout our entire lives.

Dating and Mating Are Good for You!

If you need one more good reason to get out there, learn
about yourself, and find a partner, how about this: According
to many research studies done over the past ten years, statistics

show that good relationships help you live longer, while bad relationships hurt you in many ways, including slowing the ability to recover after surgery and illness. A recent study by AARP on sexuality after age 50 reported that people with regular sex partners are healthier, less likely to experience depression and stress, and say they feel more optimistic about the future.

A lack of a significant relationship takes its toll on both sexes, but it's a little-known twist that it's frequently just as hard on a man as a woman. The myth that men are more independent simply isn't true. Older men who are not in relationships tend to be more self-destructive and are statistically more likely to die sooner than men who have partners. The reasons for this are complex. Fundamentally, older women tend to have better social and bonding skills than men, which helps them form close friendships and communities. Countless studies show that living in communities and having friends protects people from health dangers that can increase as a result of isolation.

In general, men without partners need to find loving partners in order to *live longer*, while women without partners need to find loving partners in order to *live better*. Either way, if you're single and over 50, you are more likely to live happier, healthier, and longer in a decent relationship than alone. Human beings are made to connect, relate, touch, cuddle, kiss, talk, argue, and love one another. Dating after 50 is well worth the effort to invest in your happiness—now and for later.

Like a Kid in a Candy Store

Sometimes, a recently divorced man or woman may eagerly charge out into their newfound freedom, ready to sample a bite of every new treat. This is usually an early-stage dating experience and wears off after a while. Though they may be enjoying every candy they can find, hanging out with these insatiable dessert lovers at this stage of exploration can be painful. You may want to stay clear of these early candy lovers until they've had their fill and settled down. If someone remains a serial one-night or one-month dater for months or even years, you may want to ask yourself why. Are they afraid of intimacy or do they confuse sex with intimacy? Do they have limited dating skills? Could this even be you?

One of the worst times to seriously date is when you or your date have just gotten out of a marriage or a long-term relationship. Suddenly there are no constraints and all that pent-up desire bursts through. If this is your situation, you can give yourself permission to frolic for a while, but put a time limit on it so you don't

> **Dr. Dorree Says:**
>
> I have spent more than two thirds of my life helping couples get into relationships, be in relationships, and get out of relationships. Even though relationships take work, most people simply do better together than apart.

spend the rest of your life playing the field, while actually feeling quite unsatisfied. Having fun with someone new at night, but waking up feeling detached and lonely in the morning, gets old after a while. Fishing is fun, but longer term, it's time to look for a keeper.

If you find yourself dating one of these newly paroled singles, be sure you know what you may be getting yourself into and don't delude yourself into thinking you will be able to change them before they are ready. At this early dating stage, another potential red flag is the newly separated dater who may be exceptionally needy and eager to latch on quickly to whoever will have them. Playing the role as someone's *transition object* does not necessarily lead to good matchmaking down the road. So it is wise to find out how long someone has been on the dating scene and what they have been up to. Asking these kinds of questions, tactfully, on a first or second date is not intrusive or unreasonable. Proceed with care and respect, but do proceed. After all, this is your future we're talking about.

Are You Really Too Busy to Date?

QUESTION: *I work long hours at a job I really love. My teenage kids are at my place every other weekend. I go to the movies every other Thursday with my buddies and play poker once a month, which I am not giving up. How am I going to fit finding a new partner into all this? I'm too busy to date.*

—CRAIG, 56

Many people work hard, are responsible for people other than themselves, and have full lives—and of course your obligations are important. But when it comes to dating and being fully happy in life, you need to be able to walk and chew gum at the same time. No one is too busy to date! Making time for yourself and your future sweetheart is important, so start looking for ways to free up some time in your life so you can get out there and find him or her.

Besides work and children, other excuses for not having time to date include taking care of aging parents or being overly committed to community projects, like fund-raising for a nonprofit group or volunteering. How about a little self-caring and self-generosity? Are you really so busy that you can't make time to fall in love?

No more excuses! Behind every "good reason" for not dating is a deeper reason we are keeping from ourselves. We fool ourselves into thinking we are far too busy to date when in fact we may just be afraid. More often than not, what is really going on when someone says "I just don't have time to date" is anxiety about how you look, how much you weigh, how others may see you, if anyone will really want you, and other self-confidence issues. The insecurities that plagued us as teenagers don't necessarily go away when we start dating again after 50. If anything, they can be worse. Not only have we aged and our body parts become wrinkled and droopy, we also may be less willing than when we were kids to open up and be vulnerable again.

Here's the good news: just about everyone we might potentially date probably feels just as we do! If you feel insecure about one thing or the other, odds are so does the other person. In fact, most people you date are far more worried about how *they* look to you than how you look to them.

Remember, *You* Are a Catch

Here's something fun to think about: Right this minute, people are looking for you! Someone whom you could like, maybe even love, is wondering where in the world you are. You, *just as you are right now*, are exactly who he or she would like to get to know. Stop thinking about how you have changed or what you don't like about yourself. Focus on the positive. Shifting your attention to your best features, both physical and otherwise, will make you more confident and attractive. There must be *something* you like about yourself.

Your eyes? The sound of your voice? Your quick intellect, or your sense of humor? Sure, you may have some low self-esteem issues. So does everyone else.

Many people forget that their attractiveness after 50 involves a different kind of glow than when they were young. Mistakenly, they tend to compare themselves to the image of their youth. Once self-judged as such, they are bound to lose. Most of us have a few extra pounds, sagging butts, lined skin, and look better clothed than naked. Both women and men forget that their personal attractiveness is not merely a question of physical characteristics, but a combination of many qualities: their age-appropriate looks, life skills, intelligence, hobbies, experiences, and especially their wisdom gained from these bonus years.

The scars and smiles of your years have brought you new and different qualities you didn't have when you were young. Perhaps it's your love of your children or grandchildren, your cooking, business success, golf game, easy laughter, the musical instrument you play, the knowledge you've gained from travel, or your different and possibly fuller sense of sensuality than earlier in your life. Change your perception of yourself and get out there and have fun meeting new people.

Think Pro-Aging

Though we live in a youth-oriented culture, you don't have to pretend you are young. There is nothing wrong with your body, as is, just the way nature made it. On the other hand, if there is something that you really want to change about yourself physically, and it is possible and affordable, why not? There are many procedures available today, from minor tweak-

ing with facials, hair removal, and
creative makeup, to more aggressive
transformations, such as dermato-
logical procedures, Botox, other
fine-line fillers and minor or even
major cosmetic surgery. None of it is
really necessary, but the lift you get
on the outside—while it won't solve
all your issues inside—may give you

Dr. Dorree Says:

The dating game is all
about figuring yourself out,
focusing on your best self,
and knowing what you
are looking for so you
can recognize him or her
when he or she shows up.

the confidence you need. In this competitive time of media
perfection and injected, unlined faces, it's sometimes confusing to know how you want to present yourself. On the other
hand, if au naturel is more your thing, it's wonderful to settle
into your own skin and simply be you. Remember, there are
people out there who will like you just as you are. Really!

No Guarantees

QUESTION: *I want to find a partner to share my life with, but
I don't want to sign up for a lot of problems I don't
currently have to deal with. How can I tell if the
person I'm dating is going to turn out to be more
trouble than she's worth?*

— JASON, 52

It would be great to have a dating crystal ball, wouldn't it?
All we can do is work on knowing what we want and pay
attention to what another brings to the table. If you are alert,
you can tell a lot about another person in the first hour of
meeting them, and certainly within the first several dates.

Keep in mind that no one is perfect and problem-free.
Whomever you pair with will have some less than wonderful

Dr. Dorree Says:

There are no perfect white horses; we are all spotted steeds. So choose your spots! You might as well choose someone with baggage that is a good (or at least acceptable) match for you.

personality quirks that come with his or her total package, and for sure, they won't be precisely the same ones you have. So of course you will gain a few challenges you don't currently have. On the other hand, you will also gain a whole lot of fun, happiness, and comfort you cannot create for yourself by staying alone.

By the time we hit 50, we all have baggage of one kind or another—kids, ex-spouses, emotional scars, expanding bellies, illnesses, bad habits, and we are sure you can think of a few more.

Dating Is Not a Romantic Fairy Tale

Most of us after 50 have been raised on the seductive fairy tale ideal of romantic redemption. It's hard to shake off the fantasy that Cinderella will someday be swept off her feet by Prince Charming, who happens to know exactly where to find her missing glass slipper. In real life, that fragile shoe probably broke a long time ago, and the prince is likely still a toad (perhaps with both warts and potential). Another myth: the knight in shining armor will always find his perfect Guinevere. We live in the real world, not Planet Perfect. What you are looking for is a good match, even a diamond in the rough, a comfortable partner, or some true chemistry you can't order off a menu. We are all in the process of growing as people. Part of growing up is learning to love and accept people as they really are—including yourself.

Try thinking of dating as less of a romantic quest and more

of a pragmatic task, a life project with a goal. That may seem terribly unromantic right now, but the truth is, being pragmatic at the start does not mean you can't be romantic later on. In fact, just the opposite is true. Being goal-oriented at the start will save you tons of unproductive fishing time and lead you faster to your catch.

However, the goal is *not* marriage (although dating may eventually lead to that), but rather meeting lots of people with potential and finding someone who is a good fit for you, someone you can learn from and grow with, someone with whom you can wake up in the morning and feel good about life. Later, if you want to go the next step, marriage can be explored. Love and marriage are deeply fulfilling with someone who is a good fit. Hopefully, it's not puppy love or rescue-dog love, but a real connection that can grow. After all, you probably don't want to sign up for the dating circuit again if you can help it.

Once you've decided someone is worth your time, try to look for and find the good in your partner. You don't have to marry them or even go on a second date, but cautiously focusing on the positive is a good habit to get into. Cautious optimism will keep you looking for the good while realizing there are some frogs out there. If you decide on your first date that he or she is a frog, keep in

Dr. Dorree Says:

Even if the first date is not what you hoped and you never want to see him or her again, train yourself to say an internal "thank-you" for the education he or she has provided, including helping you learn more about what you want and don't want and why you don't want it. Advanced daters can learn to shift their attitude and feel grateful for every encounter.

mind that some nice people may not have much dating experience. Even someone who is bad at dating may be good at partnering, so try to keep an open mind. Of course, the flip side is also true: some very excellent daters may make lousy partners. You may have to date someone for a while before figuring out what kind of fish you've landed.

Make a Wish List

Keep a Wish List of the general values you want in a mate and keep writing in your dating journal. What are you willing to accept? Are kids okay? Even if they still live at home? Do you want to travel a lot with someone who can afford to keep up with you? Is a little extra weight just fine if you like the rest of the package? What are your deal breakers? Is smoking unacceptable? Is religion an issue? Knowing where you draw the line can save you tons of time and heartache later.

Be careful about being too picky. Just as with house hunting, you may start out looking for your dream home with four bedrooms, three bathrooms, seven closets, and a perfect backyard, and then you suddenly find yourself falling in love with one that has only two bedrooms, no backyard, but a spectacular view in a perfect location, with a price a bit more than your budget. Stay open for new surprises when dating. All the other particulars aside, you may find that the best quality to look for in a mate is someone who is teachable and willing to grow.

Vera ended up falling in love with someone completely unexpected. Her friend fixed her up on a date with a guy who did not fit even one of her written "wish list" criteria: he had too little money, too many kids, and lived in the wrong geographical era. "But when I took one look at him, I was a goner," she says. They eventually married and are very happy.

Rating Your Dating Priorities

After you have created your dating Wish List, ask yourself:

Is my list precise and are my priorities clear?
Upside: You won't waste time with too many frogs.
Downside: You may not have left room for surprises.

Am I unsure of what I want?
Upside: You've left a lot of room for surprise.
Downside: Almost anyone will do.

Am I willing to date for fun and experience?
Upside: You can have some good times.
Downside: You may get bored after a while, and dating could wear you out.

Is marriage my only goal?
Upside: Your focus will help you to use your time and energy wisely.
Downside: You can miss out on tons of fun and growing,

Is my idea of a dream date the same as when I was young?
Upside: You will continue to dream.
Downside: As reality sets in, your dreams may easily tarnish and depression can set in.

Dating Is a Process of Self-Discovery

Before you can catch a good fish, it helps to know what you want and why you want it. Many successful daters start with a written wish list, without getting too persnickety or exacting. Checklists of priorities can save you time, but be aware that there's a fine line between having a general idea of what qualities are most important to you and creating a list that is so limiting it blinds you to a wonderful surprise that may be packaged in an unexpected way.

Mary Had a Little Man

Take Mary, for example. Divorced and alone for several years, at 67 Mary decided, with much encouragement from friends, to give dating a try. Coming from a lifetime of feeling "too tall for a woman," unattractive, and undeserving, Mary began her dating-fishing quest in the swamps, settling for weekend-only and emotionally unavailable men who ultimately did not treat her very well.

After a year of feeling disappointed, angry, and used, she dared to fess up in a group therapy session. Dr. Dorree encouraged Mary to face her long-standing pattern of choosing the same kind of date and understand why she was making these same choices in different garb. At first, Mary couldn't see how she was actively involved in ending up in unsatisfying relationships, but after a while she started to understand her role, and began experimenting with dating many different types of men.

That's when the learning really began. One group therapy session after a first date, Mary reported that she would not date a particular gentleman again because he was too short. The group was incredulous. Too short? Was that *really* the reason? Even if she didn't feel comfortable about herself with a shorter man, what was so terrible about

Dr. Dorree Says:

Left to our own devices, people have a remarkable way of following old familiar patterns hidden in new guises. Different faces, same old issues. Mature dogs can learn new dating tricks, especially with the help of a wise coach, honest friend, or good therapist in your corner.

going for a second date just to learn more about how it feels to be taller than her partner? Could it be that something else was keeping Mary from giving this guy a chance?

After many sessions and much discussion, Mary discovered that the real issue with agreeing to a second date with someone shorter than herself had a whole lot more to do with her insecurities about her own height than with him. This new insight about herself made Mary more prepared for seeing past superficial characteristics in a potential partner and more aware of what she truly wanted.

Dr. Dorree Says:

In my years of practice, I see my clients get so committed to their own growth that they rarely opt for long-term relationships with people who aren't also interested in acquiring new self knowledge and life skills.

It turned out that she actually did prefer taller men, but no longer because she needed to avoid feeling too tall, herself. At that point, Mary could confidently move on to dating someone else. With better knowledge of herself and more advanced fishing skills, now Mary knows that she likes tunas and dolphins more than minnows and eels. Catch and release dating is fine, as long as you learn as you go.

If you've had poor relationships or a harsh divorce, some counseling or therapy is probably a smart investment. Consider it the cost of going to life-learning school. Your self-esteem, as well as your sense of your sexual self, is probably a bit confused. Remember, until you change yourself, you will continue to bring your same self into every new situation. So learn as much as you can about your assets and hang-ups now so that you can enhance your wonderful qualities and change the ones that keep blocking you from the life you want and can have.

To Change or Not to Change, That Is the Question

QUESTION: *I really like this guy I've been seeing for a few months,
but he has some nasty habits that really bother me.
When can I start helping him change?*

—LEONA, 56

You can change yourself all you want, but don't expect to do a total makeover on someone else. Tweaking is always possible if the other person is open to it, but not a complete overhaul. Partners who are each working on their own personal growth typically do better than when only one person is interested in doing so.

Take a little time to think about who you are looking for. Do you want to attract an opposite or flock with a bird of a similar feather? Most couples do well when they share some general values, with some complimentary variations in personality and temperament. Imagine if you are a neat freak and you pair up with someone exactly like yourself. The two of you might end up cleaning the house for eight hours a day.

On the other hand, choosing someone who is radically unlike you or what you want in a partner, with the idea that you will change him or her later, is not a good plan. Some women may start relationships thinking they will modify their man, while men often start relationships hoping the woman won't change. Neither of these can be counted on because it's hard to custom alter another person as you see fit, and it is just as hard to stop them from changing as they naturally grow. That doesn't mean you can't share what you know with your partner and even teach him or her what you've discovered, if he or she is willing.

Consider keeping a dating journal so you can jot down a few notes after each date. This may sound cold and calculating, but it can really help organize your thinking and keep track of what could be many people over many months or longer. Think of it like a tickler system that professionals sometimes use to keep track of contacts.

Looking for Love in All the Right Places

QUESTION: *After a bitter divorce and a costly move to another city, I'm final ready to consider meeting someone new. Where in the world do I go to meet women?*

—DARNEL, 71

What an exciting adventure! You are about to learn new things about yourself as you start a new life and make new friends. One of the best ways to meet people is to go out and do things that interest *you*, not just go where you think you might find a date. When you discover activities to do and interests that spark your passion, you will have a good time, feel good about yourself, and become a more passionate lover when you find your next partner.

Here are some possibilities to get you thinking:

- Join a group or activity that allows you to feel accomplished, or try out something entirely new, such as an art class, book club, cooking class, or just-for-fun sports league.
- Volunteer at a community center, hospital, or nonprofit organization to get you out in the world, meeting people who share your interests. It's hard to avoid human contact when people are counting on you.

- Actively look for things to do. Scour the local newspapers and bulletin boards at the grocery store or churches, tag along with friends or family to their activities, or check out local college offerings (usually fairly cheap).
- Follow your real interests, not what you think you should do. As you develop more of a sense of yourself and what you enjoy, you will start to make new friends and your confidence will naturally grow. If you are a museum lover, go to museums; a cyclist, cycle; a golfer, golf. The goal is to have fun. If you happen to meet someone who shares your interests, so much the better.
- Go anywhere that has a sense of community, including churches and temples (even if you are not religious and not a member). Dating websites are also an option. And you could try Peace Corp meetings, environmental organizations, yoga classes, concerts, movie groups, sports events, even public lectures.
- Don't limit yourself to singles groups. Married people often have single friends. Network wherever you happen to be.
- Think of people from your past, such as those you went to school with or grew up with. With all the social network sites now on the Internet, their marital status is easy to find. Perhaps all that history you once shared is worth investigating again.
- Tell people you are in the market. Assure your old buddies and new friends their task is solely to introduce you to potential dates, and that they are not responsible for any outcome. This is no time to be shy or too proud. Keeping your desires a secret stops other people from helping you. Do you really want to sit home alone and have sex all by yourself for the rest of your life?

• Get out there so your new companion can find you more easily.

Like Bonnie and Clyde

QUESTION: *I am scared to death to go out by myself and try to talk to new people. What should I do?*

—CORY, 63

The solution to this common situation may be a lot easier than you think: *Find a dating buddy!* A dating buddy is a friend (of either gender) who you know and trust well enough to help each other. Going out with a good buddy makes meeting new people easier and more fun, and it gives you someone to converse with during those potentially embarrassing moments when no one else is talking much. Like the best of Bonnie and Clyde, you don't have to rob banks, but you two can join forces and fearlessly go where neither one of you might have gone on your own.

While you are out, learn how to converse with others. Most important, learn how to listen. Take your time. Nothing needs to happen overnight. If you are not one to strike up conversations with strangers in random locations, going together to singles mixers and events that are specifically set up for singles to meet can make the fishing more fun. If you feel uncomfortable, remember everyone is there for the same purpose. Don't compare your insides with other people's outsides. Even if they don't show it, they may be nervous, too. And if you don't get good vibes or the crowd is just not your type, you can always leave. That's part of what you are learning. What is your best environment? Do you prefer to fish in a pond, a lake, or an ocean? It's a good idea to decide with your dating buddy in advance how you will handle it if one of you meets someone interesting. You need your dating buddy, and your friendship is too important to be treated disrespectfully or carelessly. Discuss and agree on mutual ground rules before you venture out on your joint fishing trips.

Making the Most of the Internet and Other Dating Tools

In this age of cell phones, instant messaging, and the Internet, dating has entered a whole new era. On the one hand, finding and communicating with people has never been easier. The Internet has changed the rules and the atmospherics of dating in many profound ways. Instead of a chance meeting at the local soda shop, or a prearranged introduction at a family gathering, as was the norm generations ago, now single-and-hoping-not-to-be people log on to Internet dating websites or even social network sites to post public announcements of their availability, itemize their specific want lists, and (in some cases) reveal the most intimate details of their personal lives. Do you really want to advertise your favorite sexual positions before you even meet someone, and possibly pay for public viewing?

Interestingly, each dating website seems to have developed its own personality. Have you ever thought about what the differences are and which ones might best fit you? The website you choose is a partial reflection of you and the other people who list themselves there. Poke around for a while before deciding to join up.

When using dating websites, here are a few suggestions to consider.

- Be honest. There are some very good reasons to promote truth in advertising. Don't you want that from the dates you will consider? There is really nothing to be gained from presenting yourself as someone you are not. Who has time for that when you are trying to enhance your love life? Can you fudge a little bit? Sure. There is no perfect process.

- Be specific, but do not state more than what you are willing to have publicly known. Once something gets out on the Internet, it is permanently out of your hands, so use prudence and discretion. Think carefully before you post.

- If you use a photo, choose one that is relatively recent. If you are going to date someone, sooner or later they are going to see the real you. There is no advantage to baiting and switching.

- When first corresponding with a potential date you have met online, male or female, do not reveal your personal information, like your home address or last name. (If you remember the film *Basic Instincts*, you'll understand why.) Meet your date in a well-lit public place, preferably somewhere you are familiar with. Have a cell phone and some cash on you. Come on your own (don't let your new date pick you up), and be prepared to leave if anything feels "off." Trust your gut.

If you have the money and don't want to sort through the masses, why not turn to a professional matchmaker? But be careful they don't take you for an expensive ride. Ask for statistics on their results. If they can't or don't give them, run, don't walk to the nearest exit.

When using the Internet, paying a matchmaker, going on a blind date, or trying speed dating, be reasonably cautious but not overly paranoid. Remember, you are dating for a reason. You are interested in finding someone who is a good fit for you so you don't have to be lonely for the rest of your life and you can enjoy the pleasures of a sustained loving, sexual relationship again.

Playing It Smart: The New Rules of Dating

If you've been off the dating market for a while, a lot has changed. For one thing, in addition to the sexually transmitted diseases (STDs) we all heard about when we were young, now there is HIV/AIDS, which cannot be cured with a round of antibiotics like most STDs we grew up with So if you are going to have sex while dating, the stakes are much higher now.

With the advent of the Internet, potential bad players have a whole new arena in which to troll for victims, so you have to be alert and savvy. And if HIV/AIDS and Internet predators aren't scary enough, over-50 women and some men also face the possibility of being overtaken, mugged, or raped by someone physically stronger than themselves. Less dangerous, but still potentially painful, are the social and emotional traps we would do well to avoid. With all that in mind, here are five ways to protect your physical safety and shield you heart while dating.

Meet in a public place for the first few times. We know you've heard this many times before, but it must be restated. Do not go to someone's home, or let them into yours, until you know them much better. For a first date or even the third, joining each other for lunch, coffee, or drinks works well. You may want to avoid going out to dinner until you know you like the person. Dinner with a bore can feel like an eternity, and it's hard to get away halfway through a big meal. Consider finding a dating place that's like a home away from home. Think of it as a safe harbor away from home where you feel comfortable, such as your local restaurant, coffeehouse, or bar. Go often, get friendly with the staff, and let them in on your adventure. Make it a party and let them help you. Tell them your stories (after your date is gone) and they will laugh with you. Why do this alone?

It's not necessary to have sex or sleepovers on the first date (or even the first three dates). You don't have to rush into bed with someone you hardly know. Remember, dating is a process. Give some thought to allowing yourself the time for the process to unfold. Aren't you worth more than a lonely roll in the hay? Take your time. Ask yourself: how will I feel in the morning?

Keep your mouth zipped about previous relationships and current problems, at least until you've gotten to know each other a lot better. Men more often than women sometimes have the tendency to talk about what went wrong in their last relationship or how much they miss someone they no longer see. Neither will sweep your new date off her (or his) feet. Women sometimes reveal too much about their health problems, money troubles, or responsibilities. Both genders may indulge themselves in bashing their ex's (or even their last dates). No one likes to hear someone they just met complain about former lovers. It's easy to assume that someday you, too, could wind up in one of their bad stories. In general, everyone would do well to keep prior poor relationships and personal details to themselves, at least at the start. Do you really want to hear or tell all these tales of woe?

Decide who pays. Men are no longer expected to pay on the first date, and possibly not on any dates. Independent women may want to split the check, but even if you both want to go the traditional route with the gentleman picking up the tab, going Dutch in the beginning is often a better way to start. That way neither of you will feel obligated to the other in any way.

Think twice before lending or giving money. Loaning money to anyone changes the relationship between you for the life of the loan, and often beyond. Lending money to someone you are just starting to date sets up an uneven dynamic that you may never be able to undo. On the surface it may seem as if the person who lends the money has all the power, but quite the opposite is often true. Loaning or gifting money can be a way of paying for something (time, attention, affection, sex) you may think you cannot get for free because you unconsciously believe you are not worth it. It's not that great for the borrower, either, who may not feel as free to be authentically themselves, or may not look at you with as much respect. Even if you both can manage to dodge these potential problems, what happens if the person you are dating does not pay you back or, worse, keeps asking for more? Wouldn't you rather be his or her lover than an ATM?

Don't Get Snagged by Love Lines

Some common come-on lines to watch out for:
You're the most talented man/woman I ever met.
You're so beautiful, I can't help myself.
I'm going to leave my husband/wife when the kids are grown.
I think I love you, now let's go to bed.

My husband/wife doesn't understand me, but I know
   you do.
I'm sterile; I don't need to use condoms.
I'm so turned on, I can't think.
I've never been tested but I know I don't have an STD.
I've always been monogamous. You are the first.

Dating and Sex

QUESTION: *I found someone who really turns me on. Now what do I do?*

— ROSE, 59

Sex at the start is not necessary. There can be many rewards to taking some time to build a friendship first. On the other hand, customs regarding dating and sex have changed. "Nice girls" (and boys) do have nonmarried sex every day.

Being authentic means a man or a woman does not have to have sex just because someone else wants them to. It also means having sex when you do want to have sex, as long as your partner is willing (and you use a condom!). Either way, neither of you should feel obligated to jump through hoops. Your main obligation is to yourself. After that, you are also obligated to be real with the other person. What good is it in the long run not to be honest at the start?

Not every dating situation is on track to a long-term commitment. Sometimes people just want physical pleasure, and there's nothing wrong with that, if you are both honest with yourselves and each other. For example, an older woman dating a younger man may only be interested in connecting sexually, not building a committed relationship. Or a man may only be

---

Dr. Dorree Says:

The main thing is to be authentic with your sexuality. Today's rules differ from when you were young. Just because mother once said you shouldn't "do it" doesn't mean she's right.

---

looking for a one-night stand. For some people, sex is easier than a relationship. They like to keep score, even if they don't keep the person.

Whatever the particulars of your situation, if you are going to get sexual you might as well have fun *and* stay safe so you can really enjoy the experience.

Before you have sex, discuss the use of condoms. It can be awkward, but the subject of sexually transmitted diseases, HIV/AIDS, herpes, and the rest nowadays must be addressed. In your youth almost everything serious could be cured with penicillin. Not so today. One of the fastest growing segments of the HIV/AIDS population is people over 50. Wake up to reality. You've got to talk about it and you have to use condoms.

Women who are postmenopausal may have physical issues, such as vaginal dryness, that can be talked about and dealt with, such as with lubricants. Women may also be less sexually responsive if they have low sex hormone levels, are thinking about other things, don't like their partners, or any number of other reasons—and there's no shame in any of it.

Men, whose erections are not as hard as they once were, can have honest conversations about it *before* going to bed. Keep in mind that even men without penis problems may have trouble getting it up the first time if he is really interested in the woman and he feels there is too much riding on it. Women needn't think this is their fault. In fact, it's rather flattering!

Remember, if you are anxious about something, chances are your partner is too. Talking helps. Try starting the conversation with, "I am a little bit afraid of _____ (add your own fear here)." Admitting your fears will likely make your partner more protective of you. If not, get rid of him or her before you get hurt.

If you feel a bit anxious, there's nothing wrong with considering sex as a two-part process. Petting, making out, and foreplay do not have to include penetration, which may or may not happen at a later time. Keeping the lights off may also help you to relax.

When deciding about having sex with your date, think before you leap. At the same time, think also before you say no. You might be turning down a learning experience. Explore. You are not just learning about your potential partner, you are learning about yourself. If the issue is bad breath, say so; don't give up on the person quite yet. Stick around long enough to see where it goes. Once you know it's a waste of time, get out of Dodge fast.

Never Too Old for an STD

QUESTION: *I started seeing this really nice guy about four months ago, and I was really starting to like him, but I just found out he gave me gonorrhea! Can you believe it, at my age? I feel like a fool.*

—KATRINA, 69

No one likes to hear they picked up a sexually transmitted disease (STD). We tend to think this sort of thing only happens to teenagers and prostitutes, but of course, that's not true. STDs are passed around at every age—even to very nice people like you. That's why we say everyone, even people who don't have to worry about pregnancy, need to use condoms every time they have a sexual encounter. And furthermore, the ones that feel good are no good—meaning the lambskin condoms that slide on so smoothly and feel so good do not make good barriers against disease.

Sex without condoms is the main reason why STDs, including HIV/AIDS, are on the rise among men and women over 50. If you or your lover gets an STD, don't panic. Most can be treated quite effectively with antibiotics from your healthcare provider. Discuss everything you know, as soon as you know it, with your sexual partner. And don't automatically assume he or she has been cheating on you. Not all STDs have immediately noticeable symptoms, so your bedmate may have been infected for quite some time.

Friends with Benefits

Many of us have lost a spouse or find we actually prefer living alone, yet we crave companionship, perhaps a partner to go to the movies with, or just a trusted good buddy to hang out with. Providing it's morally acceptable and mutually agreeable, there's nothing wrong with having a good friend whom you also sleep with, with or without sex, and with or without intercourse. Friends with this extra benefit can be delightful. A special friend can keep us warm on a cold night, or comfort us when we are lonely or are simply fun to be with. Many people find these relationships are sustaining and fit *The Three Bear Rule*: not too little intimacy, not too much, but just right. Or, at least just right until one or the other of you wants something different or meets someone new who knocks your socks off. And yes, that transition can become messy. Or, as with the classic movie *When Sally Met Harry*, sometimes friendships blossom into romance.

> **Dr. Dorree Says:**
>
> I am often asked if a woman turns to another woman as she ages, does this make her a lesbian? My answer is, "No. It makes her smart."

Playing the dating game has no set rules. That leaves you free to make up your own. Just be aware that the results are unpredictable.

Women Who Tend, Befriend, and Maybe More

Statistics show that many woman, rarely men, who have never had a sexual relationship with the same gender (or at least not since the normal explorations of adolescence), find themselves later in life in a same-sex relationship. Given that with age there simply are more women than men and that good relationships keep people healthier and alive longer, these women are doing what comes naturally.

Sometimes these couples start by living together because it makes economic sense. They share their lives together, and eventually that includes sex, as well. Maybe they start out as good friends or traveling companions and one thing simply leads to another. Whatever the reasons, women who had never planned to live with or be sexual with another woman and later do so, tend to do better (healthwise and economically) than women who live alone. Many scientists believe this is due to the extra supply of the "happy" hormone, oxytocin, which flourishes when women tend and befriend.

Age Differences May Add, Subtract, or Not Count at All

QUESTION: *I like a guy almost half my age. Am I a pervert?*

—Roxanne, 51

Love makes the world go 'round, and the varieties of and reasons for attraction are endless. Although both women and men still worry about what people will think of them if they have a significant relationship or (heaven forbid) marry someone a decade or so older or younger than themselves, taboos are breaking down and individuals are finding that if they have dating experience and still fall for someone significantly older or younger than themselves, then it just might be the relationship they need.

Men have been dating younger women since the beginning of time. The most popular scenario is that of an older man, maybe in midlife, who leaves his now "dowdy" wife for a younger piece of arm candy. It's only within the last decade or so that it has become more common and out in the open for older women also to date and wed guys younger than they are. In fact, since women tend to outlive men, some therapists are using this as a rationale to encourage older women to bed and wed younger men.

Age differences have never been as fraught with so many negative implications in Europe (especially France) as they have been in the United States. The U.S. outlook seems to be catching up slowly to the European one. Without being either prurient or puritanical, one can simply favor good relationships that are based on love, honesty, and commitment. Good, sharing, growth-producing relationships are good for us, no matter what the age spread.

The fact that men who marry younger women are assumed to be seeking youth or an older woman who dates or weds a younger man is considered playing with her "boy toy" may be nothing more than a societal judgment. While there are certainly some relationships that may raise an eyebrow or two, negative generalizations about long-term committed partnerships are just a holdover from the fading past. None of us really knows what brings two people together and why they click. It is true that a committed relationship is usually easier if a couple shares common values, which may mean a similar age range, or may mean a shared religion, or may mean they have similar values about children, and so forth. But these similarities in and of themselves do not guarantee a successful long-term relationship. Whatever the relationship, to make it last joyfully requires effort. And no committed relationship or marriage can last for years without a blip here and there.

Dating Someone Else's Spouse: Morality Versus Reality

No matter what one's particular religious or moral beliefs, the real statistics about over-50s who have extramarital affairs are high. Marital dissatisfaction, long-term illnesses of a spouse, and the desire for more intimacy and sex lead many women and men to look outside their marriages for comfort, connection, sex, and excitement. Affairs with married people do happen and it can happen to you, either knowingly from the start or as a later revelation. What are your options if you find yourself tangled in this triangle?

As with everything else in the real adult world, there are no easy answers. Perhaps you didn't know she was married when you started dating and now you are emotionally attached. Or perhaps you did know from the start and didn't care at the time, but now you do. The idea that the power of your love will sweep her off her feet and permanently into your arms may be every lover's dream, but don't count on it. The cold, hard truth is that most people do not leave their spouses for their lovers. And even if you do end up together, the odds of a successful second marriage after an affair are lower than for the first marriages people are running away from.

On the other hand, supposedly happily-ever-after stories do happen. Just look at former General Electric CEO Jack Welch, who in 2002 at the age 67 left his wife to marry Harvard professor, divorcee Suzy Wetlaufer, then age 43. The couple says they are still in love and spend as much time together as possible, including raising four children.

Many other great relationships started as affairs and managed to last. So how do you decide if you stay or go? First, try to be realistic. You may want to talk it through with a trusted friend, someone who knows you well and will tell you the truth, at least as they see it. Confiding in a counselor or therapist can also be quite helpful as you sort through your feelings and options, especially if this is a recurrent pattern for you.

Being realistic may mean ending the affair, or it may mean staying, as it did for Caroline. After five years of hoping her lover would leave his wife, Caroline, 74, finally realized it was never going to happen. He had school-aged children and a full (although sexless) life with his wife. Rather than letting go of the man of her dreams, Caroline decided (with the help of her therapist) she would rather have 100 percent of his love part of the time than none at all. She understood why her man would not leave his family and found a way to be truly at peace with it.

Sometimes it's more complicated than simply deciding to stay or to go. Take Roger, for example. At 65, Roger found himself deeply in love with Becca, who at the time was in the process of filing for divorce. Before the divorce was finalized, Becca's almost ex-husband received a diagnosis of colon cancer with a poor prognosis. At Roger's urging, Becca stopped the divorce proceedings and moved back home for three years to take care of her terminally ill husband. Roger remained in the shadows but never left. Ultimately, the couple wed. This particular happy ending came about because of their shared belief that their ongoing extramarital affair was okay and that Becca's first obligation was to do the "right thing" by taking care of her husband. Would you have the desire and patience to stand by your married lover as Roger did?

Each situation is entirely unique and only you can decide what is right for you. Clearly, dating someone who is not already attached makes life far less complicated. However, if you travel this complex triangle or quadrangle path, it helps to know yourself and proceed with your eyes open.

Stay or Move On?

There is no foolproof way to know if you should continue dating someone. Using your dating journal can help you pay attention to important clues. For example, did your date call you or pick you up when he said he would? Is he or she living in the past, talking about what went wrong or what might have been? Is your date just out of a marriage and still too wounded for a new relationship? Pay attention to your gut, as well as your head. If something doesn't feel right, ask yourself why. Is it them or is it you?

You can also bring your new beau to meet trusted family and friends. They may have a more accurate perception of what is happening than you do. Choose those who have your current best interests at heart and are not living in your history or pining for "what might have been."

Be realistic about your date and yourself, including your paths not taken. By the time we get to this age, there are no perfect queens or kings. Look for someone who has the basic qualities that you want and respect. Good sexual connection or chemistry is always a plus, but don't automatically dump someone good just because the fireworks aren't there yet. Give love a chance.

Road Test

Before living together and certainly before you wed, it can be very helpful to "road test" your partner, perhaps by hitting the road. Whether it's low-cost camping or indulging in an elegant five-star trip, traveling together can put you in the fast lane for finding out:

- how money is handled.
- how relaxed you each feel out of your usual secure spaces.
- who takes the lead and who follows.
- who gets anxious doing what.
- can you make love?
- can you compromise together, or does one always get their way?
- do you like the same things?
- if there are kids involved, what do you do with them?
- who gives in?
- who is the planner?

Traveling tends to strip away our practiced facades and hastens the get-real process. Who, at this age and stage, wants to get entwined (again) if you can't enjoy being your authentic self in the company of someone you can actually get along with?

If you do travel together, it helps to pick some place that is new for both of you, not a favorite spot you used to go to with an old flame or spouse.

If you want to end it, do so kindly. If you've dated only a few times, simply tell your date it isn't working and you wish him or her the best. Longer relationships may call for more explanation, but not always. If you still like the person but don't see potential for going forward, you can tell him or her whatever you think might be helpful, but don't try to change or analyze him or her. Take responsibility for whatever is your part. And most importantly, *thank* him or her for the experience.

EIGHT

ILLNESSES, SCHMILLNESSES!
What to Do If You Are
No Longer an Acrobat

Have you ever felt like ten pounds of bad peanuts in a five-pound bag? Illness happens and life goes on, although depending upon what you've been up against, probably not quite the same as before. Sex often changes, too. When illness enters your life without a welcome mat, how eager are you to have sex if you feel sick, have physical limitations, or are in pain? And after you stop for a while, how easy is it to rekindle sex again in the future? That old expression "use it or lose it" can certainly be true.

Instead of allowing illness to steal from you a core pleasure that adds so much vitality to your years, you can use some of your well-earned life experience to find new, creative ways to enjoy sex anyway, even if you are no longer an acrobat. When life throws you an off-key note (and sooner or later it usually does), why not compose a new tune? Even with illness, sex can be your secret ingredient for making beautiful music together.

Help! My Illness Is Ruining My Sex Life!

QUESTION: *Ten years ago, I was diagnosed with chronic arthritis. It hurts when I lie on my back and I can no longer make love like I used to. At my age, maybe I shouldn't care anymore, but I miss having sex with my husband. Any suggestions?*

—RACHAEL, 59

How about starting by getting off your back and rolling over? Unless you are willing to give up sex altogether (and we hope you don't!), then something has to change to make sex pleasurable or even possible for you. Without knowing your particular likes and limitations, we can offer some general possibilities. We want to give you a new way to think about sex and a new enthusiasm for experimentation. Perhaps you can try other positions for intercourse (see Chapter 5), learn to connect more fully (see Chapter 6), or check out a new sex toy or erotic book (see Chapter 9). Maybe you will start thinking about sex and intimacy in new ways that may or may not include intercourse. Most probably the trick is not to do what has become most familiar and try something new.

Whatever you choose, please know that it is completely normal for sex to change with illness. Whether it's a chronic disease, like yours, an acute illness, recovery from surgery or a heart attack, cancer, or any other health challenge, sex is almost always impacted to some degree, either physically or emotionally, and most likely both. Even a short time away from your regular sexual activities can change how you relate sexually to your partner, perhaps even for the rest of your lives. You have many options to choose from if you are willing to have an adventurous spirit.

Satisfying Sex for Whatever Ails You

Whatever health challenges you are facing now (or may face in the future), you can still have a pleasurable sex life. Will it be the same as when you were younger or before you were ill? Highly doubtful. But with some new ideas you may not have thought of yet and the willingness to experiment just a little (or perhaps a lot), you may find that satisfying sex can prevail despite illness, and it might even be better than before.

Depending on your particular situation, what you like and don't like in bed, and what you are willing to try, you can experiment with customizing sex to fit your current condition. Remember, it's never too late for us older puppies to learn some new tricks! Here are some suggestions that have helped others with various illnesses stay sexy and connected.

Dr. Dorree Says:

Great sex for a lifetime means change and adaptation. Sex needn't die, even with or after an illness.

Communicate!

Chapter 6 is full of good ways to communicate your changing needs, concerns, and desires to your partner. No matter how close (or distant) you may be, you probably can improve your relationship and sexual satisfaction by honest conversation about each of your wishes and needs. If talking is too hard for either of you, try writing it out. It may not be easy, but it could be well worth the effort. Keep in mind that people often give what they themselves want to get. So unless you tell your partner what you want, you may not get it.

Illness requires innovation.

Has it been forever since you steamed up the windows of a car while petting heavily in the backseat? If you and your lover have gotten used to a regular sex routine (first a little of this, then move on to that) and it has now been disrupted by illness or surgery, this could be a good time to try something new. Extending foreplay and finding new ways to arouse yourself and your partner might mean returning to something you haven't done in years or getting up the nerve to try something for the first time. Look through the other chapters, especially Chapters 5 and 6, for more information and ideas.

Make love, not necessarily intercourse or even orgasm. Anything that is sexually arousing counts as sex, alone or together. If only one partner can achieve orgasm because the other is ill or injured, so be it. What's wrong with at least one of you enjoying a climax? And even if there's no orgasm for either party, the connection can still be pretty good if you both feel sexy and excited. It's all about making wise choices within the limitation of the cards you are dealt. Be creative! Necessity is the mother of invention, and conquering the challenges of illness may turn both of you into wonderful inventors.

> **Dr. Dorree Says:**
>
> Be patient and open-minded. Make it fun, gentle, and good for both of you. If you try something new and it doesn't work, so what!? Just try something else next time.

High Blood Pressure and Low Sex Drive

QUESTION: *Last year I found out I have high blood pressure and my cholesterol is bad. Could this have anything to do with why I can't get it up like I used to?*

RON, 55

Yes, there is most definitely a link. Cardiovascular disease can damage blood vessels and slow blood flow to the genitals. For women, it can prevent sufficient engorgement of the blood vessels of the vagina needed for lubrication and arousal. For men, restricted blood flow means the chambers inside the penis may not fully inflate, making your flag fly at half-mast.

Furthermore, some high blood pressure and cholesterol medications can potentially interfere with sex, causing impotence and ejaculation problems in men, uncomfortable intercourse or difficulty with orgasm in women, and lack of desire in both. Anything that slows down the physiology of the body may also slow your sex drive and ability. If you think your blood pressure medication may be putting a kink in your sex life, ask your doctor or healthcare practitioner about the many different drugs now available that might be a better fit for you.

And don't forget exercise. Almost everything you read about exercise being good for you and your heart is true. While it may not be enough to get you off medication, it can help enormously. You don't have to train for a triathlon to get the triple benefits of lower cholesterol, healthier blood pressure, and better sex. And remember, sex is exercise, too! That means making love might help you keep getting better at making love.

Sex After a Heart Attack

At 58, Dan had a massive heart attack that fortunately didn't kill him. Afterward, when Dan tried to make love, touching was good and kissing turned him on. Then he felt his heart race and he became terrified to continue toward intercourse—a common fear for many men. In fact, 25 percent of men give up sex entirely after a heart attack and another

50 percent have sex less frequently. Most of the time, such cautions are unnecessary. A study in the *Journal of the American Medical Association* concluded that a man's chances of having a second heart attack during or immediately after sex are only one in a million, so you might as well enjoy yourself. Most sexual activity puts no more demand on the heart than briskly climbing two sets of stairs.

What is far more likely for anyone after a heart attack is to become *depressed*—and giving up sex certainly won't help you much with that. Here are some tips for resuming sex after a heart attack:

- Find a time when you are relaxed and well rested.
- Take any medications you have been prescribed to use before sex.
- Cuddling and caressing without intercourse may be more comfortable to start.
- Talk to your partner about your feelings and concerns.
- Toss out the blame game for both you and your lover.

Some cautions: do not take Viagra, Levitra, or Cialis if you're taking a medication that contains nitrates (such as nitroglycerine), because the combination can cause a life-threatening drop in blood pressure. Recovery from coronary bypass surgery may require you to wait six weeks before having sex. People with unstable angina may need to abstain from sexual activity altogether. Check with your cardiologist for more information about your particular situation.

If you do take erectile dysfunction drugs, be sure to tell all your healthcare providers about it, otherwise you may end up like Jack Nicholson's character, Harry, in the 2003 film *Something's Gotta*

Give. He's a swinger trying to avoid becoming a senior citizen, and naturally he dates only very young women. But young in heart may not mean young in body. Harry is rushed to the hospital, fearing a heart attack, and is too embarrassed to admit to doctors that he takes Viagra.

Doctor: "Did you take any Viagra?"

Harry: "I don't need Viagra."

Doctor: "Positive? Because [if] I put nitroglycerine in your drip, the combination could be fatal, . . ." which causes Harry to jump off the hospital gurney and run half-naked for his life. (It's a great movie, by the way, for couples over 50 or those who are dating again.)

Walking Off Our Elevator Habit

The first elevator shaft was designed in 1853 by Elisha Otis, whose name you may recognize as it is still on many elevators. However, our elevator dependency may be a health hazard. Two additional minutes of stair climbing per day (approximately three floors) can burn more than enough calories to eliminate the average adult's annual weight gain. If you live or work in a high-rise, take advantage of the "skip-stop" technique: Walk some floors, ride some floors, walk some floors. If you live in suburbia on more than one floor, you have your very own Stairmaster. If you have none of the above, run, don't walk to your nearest gym and use the Stairmaster or buy one for home use, and remember to use it. According to a Harvard study, men who climbed more than 55 flights of stairs a week were 33 percent less likely to die than those who didn't.

Sex Despite Cancer

QUESTION: *I'm currently getting chemotherapy for colon cancer.*
Luckily, they caught it early, during a routine
colonoscopy, but the treatment is knocking me for a loop.
I barely have enough energy to get through the day, no
less make love at night. Sex is definitely out. What else
can my husband and I do to stay close in bed?

—DORRA, 71

Perhaps what you mean is "intercourse is out," because sex can continue without intercourse, without expending much energy, and even without having an orgasm. Holding each other, stroking your bodies, kissing on the lips or anywhere else, and many other ways of being physically loving can all be considered "having sex" if you feel turned on.

But if you don't feel turned on, don't beat yourself up. Cancer can be a quadruple blow to sex: the diagnosis can bring fear, depression, guilt and stress; the disease itself can cause pain and fatigue; it can hurt your body image; and the treatments often cause unwelcome side effects. We don't want to scare you, but studies indicate almost half the women who are treated for breast or gynecologic cancer have long-term sexual problems, and depending upon the type of treatment chosen, according to the Cornell University Urology Department, only 65 percent of men are able to resume sexual intercourse on Viagra, assuming there are no other drug interactions. Other studies say it's even more. If this happens to be you or someone you love, there is no reason to give in to the statistics; get practical tips and emotional therapy. It may turn the tide.

Even if *no* degree of sexual arousal is possible for you right now, you can still participate in sex with your husband. You can help stimulate him before or while he masturbates, if he enjoys that. And he can do something pleasurable for you, as well, even if it is not directly sexual, such as washing your hair (if the chemo has left you any), rubbing your tired feet, or giving you a gentle back or full-body massage, if you find that soothing. Asking your husband for something you want can give you a chance to feel how much you are loved and cherished. Showing your gratitude with a warm thank-you or a kiss is usually appreciated. And even if you just don't have the energy for any of it, simply cuddling or holding hands as you fall asleep can keep you feeling close to your guy during this difficult time.

Sex with Diabetes May Not Be So Sweet

QUESTION: *I have type 2 diabetes and occasional erectile dysfunction (ED). Will an ED drug help me?*

—WILLIAM, 48

Maybe or maybe not. Diabetes can interfere with a man's ability to get and maintain a hard erection. For about 35 to 50 percent of men with diabetes, damage to the arteries and veins interferes with the flow of blood into the penis, making it increasingly difficult to achieve and maintain an erection. This can take many months or even years to develop. Sometimes ED is the first sign that a man has diabetes.

Actually, the same thing can happen to women with diabetes, although we don't hear as much about that. Damaged blood vessels and nerves can interfere with clitoral sensation and vaginal lubrication, and cause difficulties with arousal and orgasm. In addition, high blood sugar can contribute to frequent yeast and bladder infections. Uncomfortable or painful intercourse doesn't do much to increase desire or pleasure.

Men with diabetes sometimes turn to ED medication to help them stay hard, but as we pointed out in Chapter 4, these drugs don't work a good deal of the time. Plus, no one really knows the long-term effects or how they may interact with other medications, such as those you may take for diabetes. The good news is that, with different food choices and more activity, type 2 diabetes is reversible in many people. Statistically, you probably have better odds of that working for you than only an ED drug.

Hot and Heavy

We all know it's not healthy to be overweight, but it's a myth that fat people, even very obese people, don't make love. In the real world, sex is more likely to be impeded by anxiety than adiposity. Fear of rejection, fear of not meeting the partner's expectations, and fear of not being able to perform are among the most common emotional barriers to intercourse. Overweight people suffer all these problems in spades. The body-image and social pressures they endure create numerous obstacles to sexual interaction. The most direct effect on sexuality comes from prolonged semistarvation dieting, which can seriously dampen the libido.

Fat is never stored in the penis, nor does it choke off access to the ovaries (as Hippocrates taught and generations of physicians believed), so the basic equipment required for intercourse works, even at very high weights. An item in the *New York Times*, datelined March 28, 1936, tells the world that Mrs. Gertrude Karns gave birth that day to a healthy 9-pound 3-ounce baby girl at a hospital in Shreveport, Louisiana. Mrs. Karns weighed in at 745 pounds and the father, Cliff, weighed 304.

In some cultures, being overweight is considered an asset. Men in Fiji, and other similar cultures, for example, covet obese women as a sign of prosperity. But in the U.S., highly paid and highly visible fashion models tell us thin is in. So when we carry a little extra weight, we often tend to feel we are not quite right and our body image makes us want to hide. Since putting on pounds happens more easily and taking them off becomes more difficult with age, watch your weight for health reasons, not image. Excess fat can cause serious health problems (breathing problems, high blood pressure, heart disease, diabetes, and more) that can cause you to be less active, have less sex, and be more vulnerable to illness, perhaps even shortening your life. Eating less is not always the answer. Sometimes the choice of food, when you eat it, and how active you are play bigger roles in achieving and maintaining healthy weight (see the end of this chapter for ideas).

If you and/or your partner are overweight, you may find that experimenting with some new intercourse positions, described in Chapter 5, may help you maximize closeness. If you feel self-conscious about your body, try dimming the lights or leaving on a bit of loose-fitting clothing until you feel more comfortable. And remember, sex burns calories!

Sex Despite Injuries and Pain

QUESTION: *Back when I was an athlete, I thought sex was all about my great moves. Now that I have arthritis, I'm starting to think sex is all in the joints. How can I still enjoy making love?*

—MAX, 71

We know it's hard to get in the mood for sex when you have injuries or are in pain, but did you know that the neuro-transmitters released during sex and orgasm can actually reduce pain in some people? If broken bones, arthritis, back problems, surgery, chronic pain, physical limitations (such as loss of limbs, paralysis, or wheelchair dependency), body parts made of titanium, or parts put together with nuts and bolts that need some oiling are keeping you from sexual pleasures, here are some ways to do an end run around pain so you can get back in the game.

- Take a hot bath to relax sore muscles.
- Get a massage. It helps move lymph fluids through the body, as well as soothes and stimulates.
- Create an inviting environment (see Chapter 6 for ideas for the bedroom).
- Take pain medications before sex, especially for arthritis, injuries, and postsurgery. Be careful to protect your vulnerable areas during sex, even when you feel pain-free.
- Rest ahead and plan for sex when you are not too tired. Weekend morning sex or an "afternoon delight" may make the process easier and more fun than trying at the end of the day.
- Do things that make you feel good and even sexy, such as getting your hair done, wearing a sexy negligee (or nothing at all, if you are so inclined), or if you are a guy, perhaps having a shower and a clean shave. Use clean sheets and share as many hugs as you can fit into your day.
- If you are in a wheelchair, wear clothes for easy access to your sexiness.
- Use pillows and angled wedges to make intercourse more comfortable.

- Consider getting a waterbed. Yeah, like the one you got rid of years ago because they were no longer hip—now it may soothe your hips.
- Rent funny movies together. Laughter really is healing medicine. It produces feel good hormones and reduces stress.

You can also experiment with some new moves from the suggestions in Chapter 5 that might work for your particular situation. For example, many people with arthritis

> **Dr. Dorree Says:**
>
> A flexible attitude can more than compensate for a less-than-flexible body.

in the hips, knees, or spine like to have intercourse with both parties lying on their sides. And you can also expand your sexual repertoire to include pleasures beyond intercourse.

Sex After Stroke

QUESTION: *My wife had a stroke last month and now she is partially paralyzed on the left side, including her arm and leg. I'm delighted that she joins me in still wanting to make love. I'm willing to do what it takes. What do you suggest?*

—MATT, 58

In most cases, people who have stokes are usually still just as sexual as before. When stroke hits the body on one side, it usually spares the middle, if you catch the drift. In your case, it sounds like the missionary position would work just fine, perhaps with the help of some pillows to raise her hips or prop up her legs. If she has some insecurities (who wouldn't after such a big change), be patient and kind. And if you need more touching or anything else in bed, take a look at Chapter 6 for tips on how to tell her. If you still have any body parts that work, you can still have fun!

Sex with Chronic Illness

At 51, Lori learned she had lupus. At first, the diagnosis came as a relief because it ended years of struggling to find out why she was always so tired all the time. But then the reality of having a chronic autoimmune illness began to sink in. She probably was not going to get better. Ever.

Lori joined a support group and learned new ways to enjoy her life despite being sick. But what no doctors or friends could tell her was how to get back to enjoying her sex life again. Learning to live with a chronic illness is never an easy experience. However, there actually is a plus side. For most people, knowing something is wrong and not knowing what it is is actually worse than finally receiving a correct diagnosis. Even if you dislike the diagnosis, at least you know what you're working with and can start to do something about it. In the case of a chronic illness, the diagnosis may be hard to accept, but on the plus side, these sorts of health challenges give you plenty of time to prepare, learn, experiment, and adjust so you can keep sex going. As always, creativity (Chapter 5) and communication (Chapter 6) are both key.

Statistics show that when one partner gets hit with a long-term illness, men are more likely to leave and women tend to stay and help. If

> **Dr. Dorree Says:**
>
> Women and men who care for ill partners need support from family and friends so they don't sacrifice too much and possibly get sick themselves.

your partner is staying by your side, be sure to show your appreciation and demonstrate how much you care by your actions and words. And if you are the partner who has chosen to stay and tend to your ill lover, remember not to get lost and to take care of yourself as well.

Sex with a "Stranger"

Katherine's husband was diagnosed with Alzheimer's last year and their relationship has radically changed. Now she does all the driving, manages the household, handles the bills, and takes care of endless medical appointments. Norman, 68, still gets erections and says he wants to have sex, but Katherine, 65, thinks he means just blow jobs, and she's not much in the mood now that the man she used to make love with is gone. She wonders, "How do I have sex with this new person? And what do I do about my very short fuse? I find myself screaming at him when I know he needs my patience." Eventually, this otherwise very proper lady found herself shouting at the hostess in a restaurant when they didn't have their table ready. Pushed over her limit, Katherine was utterly shocked to hear herself yell, "Another fifteen minutes?! What do you want me to do, hang around and play with myself?!" She was mortified by what she had said. But there's room for a good laugh here. When she, red-faced, managed to tell some of her girlfriends, they had only one question. "Did you get the table?"

Roles often change dramatically when a mate is ill, and pent-up anger is common. It is normal to go through a period of grieving when one of you experiences a major loss of function and the other experiences a major loss of a partnership. It's also a time of understandable confusion and perhaps some anxiety. Who will you be—and what will your sex lives be—now that the music has changed and your dance positions are different?

It may be helpful to think of your efforts to adapt your relationship and sex life to fit your new marriage as a conscious project, like remodeling your kitchen. It is not going to happen automatically; it requires thinking about what you want, what is possible, and what you are willing to try. Like any great marriage, a great sex life within a marriage takes ongoing effort. As we talked about in Chapter 6, understanding ourselves and what we want is one side of the coin; the other is learning how to communicate clearly and kindly with our partners as we change.

If you don't want to give up on sex entirely (and clearly your husband does not), our best advice to you in this difficult situation is to be creative and generous. Concentrate on your own and your partner's pleasure and on becoming a different lover. Keeping sex alive when your partner is ill often means going beyond your usual boundaries. What will you find in this new territory? Perhaps the next stage of your partnership with the man you still love, and perhaps the next stage of learning about yourself.

If all this exploring and changing is not for you, that's certainly fine, too. Just know that, depending on your beliefs and values, you do have options, including having an affair outside your marriage. People need companionship and sometimes close friendships have been known to develop into extra benefits (see Chapter 7).

Above all else, take care of yourself. Do reach out. You need an outlet and support, perhaps from friends and family, your religious affiliation, community, a support group for caretakers, or therapy—someplace you can let off steam, gain some comfort, learn new information, and not feel so alone.

You may also need help with everyday tasks. For example, Kia was reluctant to ask for help. Shyly, she told her neighbor about her husband's Parkinson's and how she could rarely leave him alone, even to shop for food. She was stunned and brought to tears when every other day someone silently dropped off a meal at her doorstep. People often want to help. Sometimes they stay away because they don't know what to do. Mentioning something specific helps people understand that they are not intruding. With the extra energy you will have, you might even feel more creative about finding ways to keep your relationship alive.

More Ways to Lose Sleep
Than You Can Count Sheep

Do you get out of bed many times at night to pee? Are you up half the night, tossing and turning? Are medications, hormone imbalances, anxiety, insomnia, restless leg syndrome, snoring, or sleep apnea keeping you or your partner awake? It's no wonder that so many of us are exhausted and sex takes a beating. A major reason one-fifth of married couples sleep separately is because one partner disturbs the other at night, often by snoring. But even if you solve snoring with a sleep study and a diagnosis of sleep apnea, who feels particularly sexy in bed with a C-Pap mask strapped to his or her face?

Cutting-edge neuroscience researchers on the brain-sleep-sex pathways are exploring new solutions for these problems.

In the meantime, here are some things you can try in your quest for rest—with a little sex on the side.

- Yoga, exercise (not at night), meditation, acupuncture, massage, and other de-stressors can be good sleep aides.
- Try sleep-soothing eating, such as no food two hours before bed and limiting caffeine during the day. Eating foods that contain tryptophan, like turkey or milk, helps release serotonin to relax you at bedtime.
- Taking magnesium an hour before bedtime can be especially effective. Very few people get enough of this essential mineral.
- Supplements containing sedative herbs, like valerian and skullcap, and/or low doses of melatonin work wonders for some people. (Please check with your healthcare provider before taking melatonin if you have depression, are bipolar, or prone to seasonal affective disorder.)
- For reasons not fully understood, we tend to have more sleep problems as we age. If you can't catch enough at night, catnaps during the day can lift your energy.

If all else fails, some people find occasional sleep medications useful. But be aware that although sleep drugs, like Ambien, Lunesta and others, are deemed nonaddictive, many people who use them feel otherwise. Plus, some people experience unwanted side effects, including sleepwalking (hide the car keys!), falling when getting up to go to the bathroom, and morning grogginess. There is also often a rebound effect, leaving the user even less able to fall asleep if you stay on the medication for too long or stop it too abruptly.

If you do end up sleeping elsewhere from your lover in order to get some rest, it's not always a negative. No one wants to make love when they are dragging. You can still keep your connection alive, even when sleeping apart, if you each maintain visiting rights that can lead to comfort and sex.

STDs Can Happen to Adults

QUESTION: *At my age, I never even considered asking my partner to wear a condom. Birth control is no longer an issue and I just assumed it was okay. Now I have gonorrhea! How could a college professor be so dumb?*

—CHRISTINA, 62

You'd be surprised how silly many otherwise smart people after 50 can be about preventing sexually transmitted diseases. It's easy to think condoms are just for birth control, which most of us are thankful we no longer have to deal with. But unless you are in a long-term, committed relationship or know for a fact that your partner does not have a sexually transmitted disease (and you are reasonably sure he or she doesn't have multiple sex partners), then condoms are a must every time you have intercourse or oral sex. When selecting condoms, remember, the ones that feel the best, work the worst. Choose condoms made from latex to effectively block the transfer of STDs.

Remember, if you happen to have an STD or genital herpes, you can still have great sex with full abandon (and responsibility). It's just another life hassle. Clearly, protection is your best friend.

Is It Physical or Psychological?

QUESTION: *I don't know if I have an illness, but I haven't been able to maintain much of an erection for about six weeks now, which is a big change for me. What's up with my penis?*

— TOM, 53

Your penis can be down for many possible reasons, and the answer may depend on who you ask. Your healthcare provider will look for possible illnesses. An endocrinologist will likely check your testosterone, thyroid, or other hormone levels. A psychologist may ask if you feel stressed, anxious, depressed, or angry. An unhappy lover might say you are too difficult to please. And a good friend might tell you to get a new lover. In reality, they may all be correct, or partially correct, or completely off base. So how do you figure it out?

If a complete medical exam (including tests for all sex hormones) rules out physical causes, your penis may be telling you something about yourself or your life that you need to know. Stress, anxiety, and depression can impact a man's ability to achieve and maintain an erection, and a woman's ability to relax and enjoy sex. For men, the sex hormones that used to kick in no matter what your stress level or emotional state may no longer guarantee you an erection after 50. Worrying about almost anything, from finances to kids, parents, relationships, career, and health, including worry about sexual performance, can shut sex down for either sex. The more you worry, the worse your performance will probably will be, and the worse your performance, the more you may worry. It can be a self-fulfilling, though unwanted prophecy.

Fear of intimacy can also block the full enjoyment of sex after 50, when declining sex hormones are not as forceful at pushing you past your fears. Like a disappearing curtain that may have been concealing some challenges all along, fading hormones can allow intimacy issues to be revealed, even many years into a long-term relationship. Anger and resentment can also be big sex killers, especially for women who may seethe with resentment for years and not enjoy sex because of it. A burst of anger in a man can directly block blood flow to his penis. And buried anger and other suppressed feelings can cause a man to lose his erection as soon as he enters his partner. (It is important to differentiate between instant loss of erection at penetration and an inability to sustain a hard-on sometime after penetration. If it is the latter, check out your physical state before you go for therapy or leave your partner.)

It's also possible that the problem is nothing more than temporary exhaustion, partner boredom, or the normal after-50 decline of hormones. Or it may be that your past years of not-so-healthy living are finally catching up with you. If so, it's never too late to turn that around (see later in the chapter for ideas).

Houston, We Have a Problem: We Have a Mopey Dick

Most men lose interest in their usual sexual activity from time to time. Total short-term loss of interest is pretty standard, while long-term loss of interest usually indicates a problem, which may be medical or emotional.

Here's a quick self-check: If you can get a midnight or morning erection or you can masturbate when you are

Houston, We Have a Problem: (cont'd)

alone, then your sometimes-hard, sometimes-soft penis is probably signaling an emotional issue, such as anxiety, depression, or relationship problems. Or you may be having an unconscious psychological reaction that makes your penis to go limp, which a therapist may be able to help you sort out.

On the other hand, if you can't get it up or keep it up when masturbating and no longer get spontaneous morning or late-night erections, then the cause is probably physical. Of course, it is also possible to have both medical *and* emotional reasons for erection difficulties. A complete checkup is a good place to start.

Mood Matters

Whether you're a tight-lipped, John Wayne type or an out-there, passionate Bette Midler, your moods do matter when it comes to sex. There are all kinds of moods that impact your sexuality. There's even a diagnosis called adjustment disorder with mixed anxiety and depressed mood, which can simply mean that there are psychological and medical terms for all mood interferences, all of which can impact your sex life—most especially depression. With added years, however, do remember this note of caution: depression can easily be confused with genuine exhaustion. Sometimes, people who have never before gotten so tired will confuse fatigue with being depressed. A simple change in schedule such as taking more naps or going to bed earlier may solve the problem. Depression *can* be both the cause and the result of sexual problems. A quick rule of thumb for judging depression is that if you have seven out of ten good days, your happiness quotient is considered pretty normal. Less than that, you may be depressed. Loss of desire can be a symptom of depression, or it may appear first and later provoke depression. A lack of interest in sex can lead to relationship problems, feelings of inadequacy, and other emotional issues, which in turn can result in depression. And of course, watch out for seasonal affective disorder (SAD). So many people are prone to winter blues. Light boxes and other aids are readily available and usually covered by insurance. Talk to your health professional if you think this impacts you.

Desire isn't the only aspect of your sexuality affected by depression. Studies show that depressed women may be less likely to have orgasms and depressed men were twice as likely to experience erectile dysfunction as those who weren't depressed. Hormones may be one of the links between depression and sex. Data from the Harvard Study of Moods and Cycles, published in 2003, revealed that women with a history of depression were 20 percent more likely to enter perimenopause sooner than their nondepressed counterparts. For the most severely depressed women, early onset of perimenopause was twice as likely. Another study described a similar effect in men: depressed men secreted lower levels of testosterone than those who were depression-free.

Besides hormone imbalances, depression can also result from illnesses, medications, the changing seasons (seasonal affective disorder), sleep deprivation, and painful life situations, such as the death of a loved one or relationship problems (situational depression). Sometimes, pushing ourselves too hard can create such physical exhaustion that we think we are depressed when, in fact, we may need to slow down and renew our energies and spirit.

Anxiety, phobias, unresolved childhood trauma, sexual abuse, addictions, and other emotional challenges can negatively affect your sex life as well. Rather than suffer in silence, consider asking your partner, friends, family members, healthcare provider, or a therapist for help. If you are living with someone who is depressed or dealing with other issues, don't walk away; talk with them, and if you get no results, pick up a phone and ask family, friends, or professionals to step in and help. They may simply be unable to be proactive about helping themselves on their own.

If you or your partner is a postmenopausal woman who feels moody and blue, hang on! Research shows that older people tend to be happier than younger people, so odds are, especially if you do something about it (see Chapter 3) you will eventually feel better.

A Prescription for Divorce?

Dr. Dorree Says:

Please ask your healthcare providers for information about every medication they prescribe, and tell each of them about all the prescription and nonprescription drugs (and even supplements) you take.

Frank and Mirabelle were fighting miserably and on the verge of calling it quits. Frank had been having a hard time maintaining an erection with his wife, and Mirabelle assumed her husband of seventeen years must been having an affair, or at least wanted to. Another woman had to be involved in some way, she thought. Why else would

Frank suddenly be so disinterested in making love?

It wasn't until the couple made a last-ditch attempt to save their marriage and sought professional help that their marriage turned around. Their therapist asked about any medications Frank might be taking. It never occurred to either spouse to ask his doctor about the potential side effects of the antidepressant he had prescribed. No one ever told them that Prozac can cause erectile dysfunction!

We're certainly not saying you should never take Prozac or other mood stabilizers, but be aware that almost all drugs and even many nonprescription medicines have side effects, can interact with each other in unexpected ways, and may negatively impact your sex life (see sidebar for details). You needn't sacrifice your sex life in order to treat depression. Some newer antidepressants are less likely to cause sexual problems, while psychotherapy (without medication) may be the answer. Do try sex first, however. It can be a great soporific (sedative) and lift the spirits, as well.

Medications Can Mess with Your Mojo

Paul was only 51, but his hairline was receding and he didn't like it one bit, so he got himself an over-the-counter remedy. The results? His hair grew, but no one told Paul that the medication might cause him to lose erections. Deciding that was too high a price to pay for good looks, Paul quickly dumped the drug. But what about all the other medications that so many of us take?

At least half of all Americans take at least one prescription drug, with one in six taking three or more medications. Five out of six people 65 and older take at least one medication and almost half take three or more. Too

Medications Can Mess with Your Mojo (cont'd)

few individuals and their healthcare providers know how all these medications can potentially interact with one another. And even fewer understand which medicines may negatively impact your sex life.

Ask your pharmacist or go online to find out the potential sex side effects of your medications. If you think a drug you're taking is hampering your sexual functioning, please do not stop taking it without talking to your doctor first. He or she may be able to adjust your dose as an aid to your treatment or switch you to another medication you may tolerate better.

Sex and Spirituality

"Oh, my God" is often uttered during peak sexual experiences and religious catharses. Some cultures interweave both ecstatic experiences. Others, such as Orthodox Judaism, have rules requiring intercourse as a primary means of ensuring that a husband and wife remain connected. For example, some sects believe that with the exception of specific holy days devoted only to worshiping God, it is the husband's duty to have enjoyable sex with his wife. Other religions consider a spiritual, sacred, or mystical experience as a subjective event where an individual makes

Dr. Dorree Says:

Medications, while potentially lifesaving for some, are not the whole story. Consider ways to create a balanced life that connects mind, body, and spiritual health.

contact with a transcendent reality and experiences an encounter or union with the divine. We can't comment on the veracity or accuracy of such reports, but we are drawn to aspects of different belief systems that consider encouraging sexual connection as important, especially when it's viewed as an aspect of the bond between loving partners.

One thing we do know with certainty is that healthy people do have and enjoy more sex, and statistics show that regular attendance at a house of worship does help keep people healthier. Controversy exists about whether or not this health boost is due to the power of prayer, touching a "spirit" or energy force beyond what we see, or simply the real power of community contact to improve health. Whatever your personal beliefs, we urge you to do what you can to stay healthy, connected, and if possible, be in a loving relationship. (If your relationship needs help, see Chapter 6, and if you don't currently have a partner, see Chapter 7.)

Someday, the vow "in sickness and in health" may apply to you. At such times, be sure to use whatever life skills and beliefs suit you.

Be Your Best Sex-Health Advocate

Beth had a terrible rash that was spreading across her whole body. Itchy and alarmed, she naturally ran to her primary care doctor, who was at a complete loss about the cause. He asked her about the foods she had eaten recently or any bug bites or a change in laundry detergent. Stumped, he sent her home untreated.

After days of suffering, Beth came up with a question for her physician and the diagnosis was obvious. Her husband had

developed an infection on his penis, and two days after intercourse, Beth started to itch. Antibiotics quickly cured them
both. The treatment would have helped much sooner, but it
just never occurred to Beth's physician to ask a 69-year-old
woman about sex.

When it comes to sex and health, you can get as many different opinions as there are health practitioners out there. No
one approach or person knows all. Sometimes finding the
right fit seems as complex and unwanted as the dating game.
But after all, this is your health and sex life, so it's worth the
effort to get the answers you seek.

The way medicine is practiced is rapidly changing. New dis-
coveries come every day. Politically, economically, and healthwise, prevention is in. Over-the-counter self-care is in. Local
pharmacies, supermarkets, and compounding pharmacies (ones
that custom-mix prescriptions and often use more biofriendly
medicines) are all responding to the public's increasing interest
in alternative treatments. According to the Centers for Disease
Control and Prevention, at least a third of American adults
now use alternative medicine, including acupuncture, nutritional supplements, chiropractic care, and much more. Even
the Harvard Medical School frequently encourages doctors
and their patients to seek alternative treatments.

Mainstream medications often interact with one another,
sometimes causing as many problems as they cure, especially
dampening one's libido. How can someone like Jill, who takes
forty-two medications daily (we're not making this up), possibly
know which one is doing what to her, or why she feels so tired
all the time and has no energy for a relationship, no less sex?

Self-education is your best ally. Think out of the box. Be

willing to explore and learn to trust your own body. Read books, talk to friends, interview doctors, and research the Internet. If the computer is not your friend, ask for help. Perhaps your kids or grandkids can help you. (In today's fast-changing world, the younger they are, the more adept they are with technology.) Use the Web for information, but cast a skeptical eye.

This is your life. Take charge. And if you are too sick to take charge, turn to your partner, a friend, or even a patient advocate (check your local hospital).

Healthier Is Sexier!

QUESTION: *I like having sex with my wife, but to tell you the truth I get easily winded when we make love and I feel exhausted the next day. I know I've put on too much weight and the beer and cigarettes aren't helping. How can I get back the old me in the bedroom without spending all day in the gym?*

—ROCCO, 57

You've probably had enough lecturing for the rest of your life about the many health benefits of quitting smoking, losing weight, and exercising, and you probably feel crummy about the countless New Years' resolutions you haven't kept. We know you've heard it all many times before. You can't get through a single day without the TV, magazines, doctors, celebrities, nagging family members, and every ad for some new diet or gym proclaiming you should eat right and shape up. But what good do all the constant blah, blah, blah's about diet and exercise really do? Despite all the health information out there, more than 60 percent of Americans are overweight and at least 30 percent are dangerously obese, according to the National Center for Health Statistics. Some studies indicate the numbers may be even higher. The U.S. Surgeon General's office says that obesity kills at least 300,000 Americans each year—that's more than 800 people a day dying from being fat.

Clearly, the message isn't getting through.

So let's skip the same old story about diet and exercise and focus on what matters to you, which is having great sex with your wife (or husband). Want better sex? Change your day! Whatever your general physical condition or specific health challenges, *anything* you can do to improve your health each day will contribute to having better sex, alone or with a partner. This includes exercise of any kind, watching what you eat, and making sure you have some downtime. Getting help on the cigarette and beer issues would be wise, too. Sound impossible? With effort maybe the rewards will make it worth it to you. Even the tiniest health improvements can have big rewards.

Start Now, Start Small

You don't have to wait until you have the right exercise equipment, perfect diet plan, all the right foods, or a gym membership to get started. You can begin simply by going outside and taking a deep breath of fresh air, if you can. Or go through your kitchen and start throwing out (or giving away) all the items you know aren't good for you. Or park your car a little farther away than usual and walk a bit more. Even a relaxing bath counts as healthy foreplay as you start the process of creating the new and improved you.

If you spend any time or money on external tweaking (hair, nails, maybe even a little nip and tuck), why not also do a bit of internal tweaking? If you haven't done much for your health in a while, don't worry about it, that's all in the past. Each day, begin anew. Start with small steps and build as you go. And of course, check with your healthcare provider if you have any illnesses or health conditions.

Stress Less for the Best Sex

When we were younger, our bodies were on the "stress now, pay later" plan. Now, "later" has come and the stressors of the past—too little sleep, poor nutrition, smoking, drinking too much, recreational drugs, inactivity, pent-up anger, overdrive careers, unprotected sex, or just plain self-neglect—may be starting to catch up with us. On top of that, any additional stress we might be adding today may become a "pay as you go" proposition, with an immediate price tag. Our older body parts and organs cannot roll with the punches as quickly as they once did.

At any age and with any illness, *now* is a good time to consider moving past some of your habitual stressors and putting yourself at the top of your list. If you don't have an illness, a healthy body will help you prevent one. If you have an illness, building and protecting your health can keep your illness from progressing as quickly. And even if you have twelve illnesses, taking care of yourself now may help you from getting number thirteen later.

Great sex after 50 comes in part from taking care of yourself, eliminating or reducing the stressors that tear you down, and adding more of what builds you up—like good food and more movement. We hate to tell you this, but ultimately, there is no one who can do it for you. If it's too hard to get started alone, find a buddy who can do it with you.

Good Food for Good Sex

We are not going to tell you what foods to eat. We believe green is good. However, some who live long never touch the stuff and there are plenty of cultures that eat, drink, and be merry and somehow stay healthy while they're doing it. Their foods are mostly unprocessed and they tend to eat them in moderation. On the whole, America's fast food diets seem to be health killers. But no one diet is right for everyone. Pay attention to what you do eat.

Some foods are considered aphrodisiacs. For example, there is some evidence that:

- **Chili peppers** heat up the bedroom by triggering feel-good endorphins.
- **Chocolate**, while not great for the waistline, is rich in the amino acid phenylethylamine, the "love chemical" that serves as a natural antidepressant.
- **Pine nuts** and **oysters** are both rich in zinc, which is necessary for sperm production.
- **Tomatoes**, dubbed in Italy as "love apples," are packed with lycopene, known for being a libido enhancer. (Lycopene improves eyesight, too, which also can be sexy.)

Move That Sexy Body

Everyone needs exercise. Ideally, a good combination of strength exercise (weights or Pilates—strengthening your front core—keeps your back strong), cardio exercise (brisk walking, swimming, running, or dancing) and flexibility exercise (stretching or yoga) is best, but any movement is good. Pick what you like, but keep in mind that the one you dislike the most might be your "must do." Interestingly, men often benefit most from the very exercise they resist or consider "airy fairy," like yoga or Pilates. And women tend to shy away from lifting weights or strength-building, and from movement-oriented martial arts like karate, judo, and qigong, which they typically need most. Sometimes both men and women fool themselves into thinking if they just take enough fancy vitamins, they don't need exercise at all. Nutritional supplements can be great, but vitamins that aren't metabolized result in nothing but expensive urine, which is not going to build the muscle strength and bone density we all need after 50.

You don't have to spend money to get fit. Make it easy on yourself by pairing up with an exercise buddy, or follow along with a TV exercise program, or in this Internet age, participate in a free exercise class on the Web. And don't forget: sex is exercise, too!

How much would you be willing to give at the end of your life for just one more year or even one more night with the person you love? A day at a time, starting today, healthy lifestyle choices, good food, and more movement are the ways we can extend our lives, prevent or postpone illness, and gradually build the strength we need to have the best sex and lives possible. And no matter what illnesses may slow us down along the way, there are always creative ways to have sex, even great sex, all the days of our lives.

A Final World on Illness and Sex

Let's get real: illness sucks! Even if you don't get hit with one of the biggies, like heart disease, cancer, or stroke, all sorts of other things happen that can mess with sex, like prostate problems, vaginal illnesses, urethra leaks, vaginal prolapses, men's breasts that grow, women's breasts that shrink or go flat, nipples that become less sensitive, limp penises, and low libidos from dozens of different causes.

So what can we do? How about saying, "No way will I let (insert name of illness or injury) take away *all* my fun!" If you have any part of you that can still move and feel, if you have a partner or even if you don't, if you can think even one sexy thought, you can still have sex. It may be hard to let go of past expectations and accept what is now possible, but once you do, whole new sexy possibilities can open up for you.

NINE

THE GREAT JOY RIDE
Something Fun for Everyone

Psssst. Wanna know a secret?

Grownups, even some very grownup grownups, are playing . . . with sex toys! In fact, for couples and singles alike, there is a revolution occurring for people over 50. Adult sex toys, pornography, erotic literature, game playing, and other pleasure products and practices have become much more mainstream than ever before. This is good news for those in good health because sex toys can add fun and excitement to adult life. And it's even better news for those in ill health because there are many new products available to help make sex easier, possible, and more satisfying for those with health challenges—like eyeglasses and hearing aids for the bed.

You're Never Too Old to Play with Toys

Whatever your situation or age, jazzing up your sex life with sex toys and perhaps pornography can be a great way to feel vitally alive and sexy for all your years. Single folks may find that a little help from a manufactured friend, like a vibrator or other sex toy, can be a welcome addition. And for couples in long-term relationships, some added spice is always nice. While no sex gadget can fix a broken relationship, experimenting with sex toys, porn (his, hers, and for couples), erotic books, educational sex films, role playing, and perhaps even working with a sex or relationship therapist, can be very helpful for lifting an otherwise good relationship out of a passion slump.

Dr. Dorree Says:

Anything that is mutually desired between adults who trust each other is okay. The key words are trust and mutual desire.

Wake-Up Call

QUESTION: *My wife never complains, but for the last few years, sex has gotten pretty dull. We get along better than in most marriages I know, but lately I feel more like a sleeping partner than a lover. How can we reawaken the passion in bed?*

—EDUARDO, 64

Have you wondered if maybe your wife is as bored as you are? Marriage is wonderful in many ways, but anyone who says it never gets dull in the bedroom probably hasn't been married for very long. The more years you spend together, the more you may enjoy the benefits of adding a little heat to your love life. It's hard for most couples to maintain a close connection without conversation and physical contact, so the sooner you get back to the passion, the better. Good sex, like most things in life, takes a little forethought and effort—but we wouldn't exactly call it work!

One option for taking your relationship to the next stage of intimacy is to talk with your partner (away from the bedroom; see Chapter 6) about some things that each of you may want to try. Maybe reveal a fantasy you haven't shared yet or suggest a game you'd like to play. Or perhaps introduce the possibility of trying some new sex toys or props.

Consenting adults are free to go as far (or not as far) as they please. This can include feathers, vibrators, dildos, blindfolds, whips, chains, ropes, even hanging from the ceiling if one's older bones can safely handle it. Or you can customize your sexual experiences with costumes, role playing, and fetish items, like handcuffs or super–high high heels if that happens to be your thing.

If one or both of you are not the particularly adventurous type, perhaps all you need is some soft candlelight and a bottle of bath oil, lotion, or lubricant. Remember, this is supposed to be fun, not terrifying or uncomfortable. There are plenty of ways to feel close without going too far out on a limb (like tantric sex, for example). Whatever brings you pleasure, is safe, and takes you out of the ho-hum is good.

Vibrators: Get Your Buzz On

QUESTION: *I've been secretly using a vibrator for years, usually when my husband is out of town, or at least out of the bedroom. Lately, I've been longing to include the vibrator in our lovemaking, but I don't want him to think less of me. How can I bring this up?*

—RITA, 72

Why would your husband think less of you for enjoying a vibrator? Maybe he would like to use it, too. (Maybe he already does!) Did you know that nearly half of men and 53 percent of woman say they use vibrators, according to a study published in the *Journal of Sexual Medicine* in 2009? And vibrators are not just for masturbating. Researchers at Indiana University surveyed more than 3,000 mostly heterosexual adults in 2008 and discovered that, among people who say they use a vibrator, 81 percent of women and 91 percent of men reported enjoying it with a partner. In fact, according to two separate studies, vibrator use is associated with more positive sexual function and being more proactive in caring for one's sexual health.

No longer just a solo act, sex with vibrators has come of age. Once considered merely a temporary tool to help "sexually dysfunctional females" achieve orgasm (as reported in the *Journal of Popular Culture* back in 1974), today's vibrators are as common in American bedrooms as coffee pots in our kitchens. And rather than having to buy a vibrator in the back room of some adult sex store or through the mail in a plain paper wrapper, now you can grab one right off the shelves at Sharper Image, Walmart, Walgreens, CVS, and both high-end and inexpensive department stores—in fact, at almost any mall. Even easier, you can buy online. At www.Fiftyand Furthermore.com, Dr. Dorree recommends vibrators that she thinks are great. Or for an even wider selection, www.amazon. com has a Sexual Wellness store with more than at least 25,000 items, and countless other legitimate non-porn websites abound.

Vibrators can be fun, inexpensive, easy to use, portable (take it on vacation!), and best of all good for you. All forms of sex, with or without orgasm, are healthy (assuming your heart can handle it). And getting your buzz on with a vibrator promotes positive sexual function at every age.

So the next time you are headed for bed with your husband, if you think he will take it well, try leaving your secret pleasure toy out in the open, perhaps on his pillow, perhaps with a love note, and see what happens. Or if you suspect a vibrator surprise might be seen as a negative message, you could have a conversation with him about it first to relieve any anxiety either of you may be feeling. Remember, this is your life partner. He can probably handle the truth about what you really want, and in any case, this is your time to be your true and authentic self, while keeping what is best for your relationship in mind.

The Joys of Toys After 50

While vibrators are the most popular after-50 sex toy, there are many other passion playthings on the market today. Over 50 is the perfect time to incorporate adventure (and convenience) into your sex life. After all these years, we've finally arrived at the joys of sex unzipped. In the privacy of our own homes or hotel rooms, alone or with our partners, no one is watching or keeping score. Adults over 50 are grown up enough to enjoy their sex lives to the fullest, and they are going for it in droves.

Researchers attribute the widespread use of adult sex toys to easier availability and a cultural shift away from the bad boy, triple-X-rated sex toy industry. New Internet sites for sex products aimed at mainstream couples now feature images of middle-aged models and realistic sex scenes. Women are buying more sex toys and pleasure products than ever before—

which hasn't gone unnoticed by the adult novelties industry. In fact, several companies now market exclusively to women as young as sorority sisters and as old as postmenopausal golden girls. In many regions of the country Tupperware-type parties have given way to adult toy sales gatherings, almost always attended and led by women.

Not only are women buying and using more sex toys, the sales of erotic novels are up, too, even in a down economy. An entire flourishing industry now markets erotica especially for women, including older women.

Finding What Works for You

QUESTION: *A couple of days ago, I went into an adult sex shop for the first time and I was so confused that all I could do was make a quick lap around the store and get out of there as fast as I could. How in the world do I know what I want?*

—ERICA, 65

First forays into adult sex stores can be embarrassing and even intimidating, but going online and shifting through the gazillions of mostly useless and often expensive sex products can also be pretty overwhelming. One is better off seeking the advice of a trusted friend or a knowledgeable sex educator. If you can screw up your courage to ask for help (we understand it may be too hard), salespeople in adult sex stores are like good salespeople in all stores. They usually know their products and enjoy their work. If that's too embarrassing, Dr. Dorree sug-gests going to a knowledgeable therapist and educator, like herself or one of her well-trained colleagues. Gadgets are fun and can enhance your love life, solo or together, but as with all products, selecting what best suits your needs often takes some sage advice.

Women tend to purchase online to maintain privacy, though they often think nothing of paying by credit card. Men, not surprisingly, like to see and touch what they buy, and are less shy about going into brick and mortar stores to survey the goods and ask questions. Either way, there is a wide range of prices for the same items and some have huge markups. It is best to purchase items from someone who is very familiar with their pluses and minuses. The end user (you!) has to be aware of any potential negative side effects.

Remember, these toys are for your pleasure, so it makes sense to get items that will be easy to use, feel great, and get the job done. While younger people tend to focus more on how snazzy a sex toy looks, more mature types like to feel good about using it and want to get the most benefit from it—like the ability to be aroused quickly and easily so we can enjoy our partners and still have time for a good night's sleep.

And why not? If we can use eyeglasses, hearing aids, canes, dentures, large-size type, wheelchairs, support stockings, knee braces, orthopedic shoes, wigs, push-up bras, vitamins, sun block, Botox, glue-on fingernails, false eyelashes, back supports, and all manner of other technologies to make our lives work better, why in the world can't we use sex-enhancing technologies in bed? This isn't dirty or shameful; it's stimulating, fun, and makes sex less physically demanding. For adults from 50 to 100, sex toys make sex a lot easier, and for some, even possible.

Talk about coming out of the closet. Not all sex toys are made to be solely utilitarian. Some are now being created as objects of art that can be proudly displayed for all to see (if you happen to be so inclined). For example, Lelo is a Sweden-based company committed to designing what they call "sensual pleasure objects" that combine fashion, femininity, and functionality in visually pleasing sex toys. Some are sculpted out of special nonbreakable glass into beautiful art objects, with art prices to match. Yes, the world has changed from when we were growing up. Sex is not so under the covers or even between the sheets, but truly out in the open for many adults.

What People Buy and Use

Women and men from age 50 to 80 and beyond tend to be very specific about what sex products they purchase. Although some will buy (and use) almost anything available, most gravitate toward more functional and natural items that may make their daily lives a bit more joyful and easy. Interestingly, older people are more likely to purchase more ecologically green sex-enhancement products than younger buyers. It's nice to think we are still doing our part to protect the planet, even when we're getting our rocks off.

As we age, our bodies need more care. Lubricants, or lubes as they are known in the trade, help counteract vaginal dryness, prevent too much painful friction on thinning vaginal walls, and help the penis (or dildo) glide better. Women tend to do best with lubes that help maintain the natural pH balance of the vagina, protecting it from irritation and infection.

Mature women tend to purchase vibrators for external clitoral stimulation and may shy away from internal vibrating dildos or vibrators with too many bells and whistles. Both men and women like vibrators for clitoral stimulation because older bodies sometimes tire more easily, and when foreplay isn't working or is taking too long, or one or both of you are getting tired, a clit stimulator can usually put her in a state of arousal (and even orgasm) fairly quickly.

Older women (and men) also like dildos with the look and feel of the real thing, as opposed to younger buyers who often go for rock-hard, multicolored, or electronic dildos. Older women like to hold their dildo in their hand (or have their partner hold it), which gives them more control. Newfangled dildos that move or make noise are harder for stiff fingers to control and can be intimidating. In general, those over 50 tend to stay with what they are already familiar with. (In case you may be wondering, a dildo is anything shaped like a penis that can be inserted into any orifice. A dildo may or may not vibrate. A vibrator is anything that vibrates, and may or may not also be a dildo.)

Certainly, older men want to keep their erections going. If they cannot take erectile dysfunction (ED) pills or are wisely wary of them, they like sex-enhancement items that can help keep an erection up for as long as possible. One of the most popular choices is still the old reliable cock ring. Variations of the cock ring have been around forever, but with our new sexual freedom and the development of more user-friendly materials, there has been a surge in their use. Most men over 50 are on one medication or another, and the nonpharmaceutical cock ring can be an excellent choice for maximizing a hard-on without risking any drug interactions. The safe, low-tech cock ring delivers the results men want and can easily be used with condoms.

There are countless herbal formulas, love potions, and other products that are supposed to enhance sex for men and for women, but be very leery of anything to be taken internally that has not been approved by the FDA, no matter how good they sound. For example, there are products with wonderfully sexy names like "Male Verility" and "Rock Star" that sound oh-so seductive. But unless you know exactly what they are made of and how they may affect you or interact with medicines you are already taking, stay away. Besides being potentially dangerous, these sex potions do not work for men who are totally impotent. The ones that can work are those that help enhance and prolong those softer erections that naturally come with age.

Pet Shop Toys and Other Sexy Bargains

There are hundreds of thousands of sex toys on the market today and some of them are pretty darn pricey—even ridiculously so. With a little creativity and fun, you can come up with all kinds of less costly alternatives that are just as good, maybe even better. Here are some ideas to get you started.

- Do you like the idea of a doggie collar and leash for yourself or your partner? Why spend oodles of money on rhinestone-embellished or metal-studded collars and other goodies when you can save money at your neighborhood pet shop? A fun trip through the pet supplies center, alone or with your lover, can be an exciting experience as you pick out plenty of perfectly good stuff for much less than in the sex stores—and no one there will know what you are up to.
- Investing in a good vibrator will bring you years of fun and service, but if you just can't get one, try an electric tooth brush instead (use the handle end only, *not* the brush!).

- Pop open a household pillow for flirty feathers that you can tie to a string and dangle across your lover's skin.
- Skip the costly fruit-flavored lotions and raid your refrigerator or pantry for fruit you can throw in the blender and pour on yourself or your partner. (But keep away from the genitals. Sugar, unless totally licked off, can cause yeast and urinary tract infections. Why take the chance?)
- For those truly adventurous types, most foods that don't contain sugar or citrus (acid-based) can be eaten from several orifices. Use foods that go from warm (not hot) to cool (not cold).
- A little whip cream can be fun, too.
- One connoisseur of oral sex swears that the only problem he ever had with oysters was that they tended to get lost and were hard to find.
- Ice cubes on testicles and nipples in moments of passion are an old standby for extra stimulation.
- Some swear by Alka-Seltzer, which snaps, crackles, and pops when inserted into the vagina. Users claim this alternative method temporarily cures dull sex as well as the more common upset stomach, acid indigestion, and headaches.
- Alcohol, especially champagne, is often tempting. But remember, alcohol burns and champagne, though in fantasy remains romantic, is still alcohol.
- Use old belts and scarves instead of pricey handcuffs and restraints. (Use only with a consenting partner, and be careful not to fasten too tightly).
- Consider keeping a pair of those four-inch stilettos that you can no longer walk in. Keep a pair for bed fun fantasy. They don't hurt when you are lying down."

Lube Job

QUESTION: *I keep seeing TV ads for "tingling" sexual lubricants for women. Are these safe to use?*

—JACLYN, 75

Maybe, but probably not. Most women over 50 tend to dislike "warming" gels. Cautious use is wise. As with all additives, read the label. Some products that feel good aren't. For example, many warming jells contain methane which under other conditions is a combustible gas. No one wants that kind of fire on or in his or her body. For the same reason steer clear of unknown products that tingle. A brief moment of fun is certainly not worth possible long-term damage. Again, older people tend to like things that are more familiar and natural. Still, if you find the idea intriguing, and you know it's safe, why not give it a try?

Just be careful that you don't end up like poor Lisa. One night while making love, Lisa's husband of twenty-seven years decided, in a rare creative moment, to use a common household product, Noxzema, as a surprise stimulant to give his wife an extra boost. And what a boost it turned out to be! Lisa, 62, shot out of the bed and into the shower and then into the bathtub faster than a rabbit with its tail on fire. Noxzema can burn the sensitive tissues of a woman's vagina like the sting of a thousand bees. Lisa was angry for days and her husband vowed never to spring a surprise on her again—a good promise for any couple to make. Guys, too, suffer from thoughtless surprises. Bill's wife once surprised him with a sip of cognac in her mouth during a blow job. He, like Lisa, spent forever under the shower and in a tub. Their household was not a happy place for either partner for over a week.

Save the surprises for birthday gifts and discuss any product you may wish to use in bed to be sure it isn't something you may be allergic to, or that could cause unanticipated, even painful side effects. Some products carry labels that warn you to avoid use if you have sensitive skin, are pregnant, or have dormant herpes that may become reactivated.

Making the Most of Male Masturbators

QUESTION: *I've been alone since my wife died four years ago. At 78, I don't expect to ever have a sex partner again. I do masturbate almost every day, but honestly, sometimes it's just too much work. I'd love to have an easier way. Any ideas?*

—DARSHAWN, 78

Did you know that after 50, there are about ten single women for every four single men? And all you need is one. At 78, you still have a lot of life to enjoy, including the very real possibility of a future love life (check out Chapter 7). But on to your question about easier masturbation.

Some men find they enjoy a masturbation sleeve in which you insert your penis with some lubrication and slide it over your erection to feel somewhat like a vagina. Even in a relationship, using a male masturbation sleeve may bring you both excitement and joy. And it may come in handy if one of you is just too tired for sex after spending the day running after grandchildren, but doesn't want to let your loved one down.

For some men, especially those who are single, a sleeve just isn't enough. They may miss the feel of a body pressed against theirs and want something more substantial to hold. For them, a masturbator sex doll can be helpful. These come in many sizes, shapes, and costs, ranging from a relatively inexpensive inflatable to a high-end, very humanlike, full-size sex doll, complete with realistic features—like eyelashes, breasts, nipples, and a functional vagina. If you are a more adventuresome type, a sex doll may be a fun addition even with a partner. In other cultures sex dolls are more openly accepted. An estimated 10 percent of men in Japan openly take their life-size dolls to dinner with them. In the U.S., many may find such openness hard to accept, and though we are not promoting the idea, we can certainly see how it eliminates the need for couple's therapy!

Senior Sex

Folks in their 70s, 80s, and beyond buy sex toys, too. With increasing age, most people prefer nonelectric dildos to things that go bump in the night, make odd noises, or move strangely. They also prefer vibrators that are lightweight, quiet, and easy for fragile arms to hold and control.

For those who don't like traditional vibrators, the Jack Rabbit may be handy. Created in Japan over twenty-five years ago, this unique "twice as nice" vibrator claims to be the first to offer simultaneous stimulation of both the inside of the vagina and the outside of the clitoris. With its unique design and variable speed control, the Jack Rabbit has popped up on numerous TV shows, including a cameo appearance in 1998 on the HBO hit series *Sex and the City*.

The masturbator sleeve (discussed earlier) can also be helpful for arthritic fingers that just can't do what they once did or when, perhaps, dental issues (such as false teeth) possibly interfere with oral sex. With a sleeve, no one has to grip hard, and both partners can participate together. Even if she's half asleep, he can put her hand on his (or vice versa) and guide her. Sex becomes a mutually satisfying experience as well as easy on the body.

Many older couples have learned to use sex aids while having intercourse. Life is easier, no one has to work as hard to achieve orgasm, and sex is still fulfilling and intimacy is sustained. Pretty cool, isn't it?

Some externally applied creams can be helpful, too. Both clitoris and penis engorge when blood flows to the region, which leads to expulsion of the extra blood and creates an orgasm. Therefore, topical creams that aren't absorbed into the body and don't interfere with blood flow are best.

There are also creams that do get absorbed and have an internal effect of some kind over time—or at least their manufacturers say they do—and some people swear by them, although there currently are no scientific studies proving their effectiveness. Because these topical creams, usually applied to the genitals, are absorbed into the body over time, one is wise to be cautious and make sure there will be no irritation or other adverse short- or long-term effect. It is especially important to know the ingredients of these creams and their possible interactions with any pharmaceuticals or over-the-counter herbs that you may also be using for other purposes. Read ingredients and stick to water-based lubricants. They remain the safest.

Conquering Challenges with Sex Toys and Fantasies

Genine came from a solid Baptist home. In fact, her father was a preacher and sex was never talked about or even alluded to in any context other than procreation. After thirty-two years of marriage and three almost-grown children, Genine is just now learning how to masturbate. Her husband can no longer have intercourse because of a medical problem. The couple can kiss and hug, even give each other massages, but they have to stop their sexual contact before he gets too aroused. At 61, Genine uses porn videos and various vibrators to have sex by herself, away from her husband. Genine says she often fantasizes about other men and has had many opportunities to experiment with others, but she would rather have the joys she shares with her husband than go elsewhere. Sex toys have become her friends.

Maxwell, 72, is a highly competent electrical engineer who is still a powerhouse at work and a loving husband at home. Three years ago, his penis stopped working entirely and erections became impossible. Rather than feeling inadequate and giving up sex, Maxwell snaps on his very own "ménage a trois" dildo and uses it to pleasure his wife. While he can no longer have orgasms himself, it gives him great satisfaction to continue to give to his lover and to see her satisfied.

Kathy, 78, has a recurrent fantasy. A real bad boy, loaded with tattoos and in full motorcycle regalia, pushes her to the ground, mounts her like a dirt bike, and thrusts his hard penis deep inside her. Kathy, who says she was brought up "proper" and has never strayed from her 54-year-old marriage, feels no guilt using this fantasy with her accountant husband most every time they have sex. It's her secret pleasure.

Lori, 59, thinks she's found a powerful sex potion called

pheromones. Although pheromones are naturally secreted by the body and are believed to impact sexual attraction, so far there is little scientific evidence that the manufactured ones actually work. In fact, they may only have a placebo effect. But many people believe they do attract the opposite sex. Some worry that every

> **Dr. Dorree Says:**
>
> Grownups don't need to follow old rules. We are perfectly capable of making up our own rules, as long as they are safe and mutually agreeable.

human, dog, and cat will follow them home, while others wish it was true. Either way, Lori is happy. She feels sexy when she dabs on the liquid and is more likely to flirt for the rest of the day. Do pheromones work? Lori has more confidence and projects a sexier self when she uses them. Someday, science will know more. For now, it's working for Lori.

George, 71, and Hilda, 69, have been married for forty years. Not big fans of sex toys or high-tech gadgets, the couple was mired in bedroom boredom for years until they discovered the simple joys of a sexy board game that directed them to answer revealing questions and disclose fantasies to each other every time they had sex. That's all they needed to get their love lights shining again. After a few months the game ran its course, and George and Hilda decided to try something new once a week—like making love in a new place in the house, or enjoying the unique sensations of various household items, such as whipped cream, strawberries, and even ice cubes.

Pornography: His, Hers, and for Couples

For years, women barely tolerated male pornography, although some would sneak a look at *Playboy* or *Penthouse* themselves. Men, more than women, tend to have a very strong visual component to their sexual arousal and they are more likely to seek visual pornography to get turned on. Pornography can be a wonderful sex enhancer for both men and women, but there is a difference between enjoying some fun porn and being addicted to pornography or engaging in potentially dangerous sexual encounters—both of which are now easily available on the Internet. Addictive porn and dangerous sex almost always hinder loving sexuality and intimacy. Women typically enjoy a different kind of porn than do men, usually with characters and a story line. Female erotic literature has become a booming business, and it is one more example of how women, who are generally the less linear of the two sexes, prefer process over the end goal. Not that women don't like to see or read about orgasms. It's just that women more than men tend to get turned on by what *leads up to* sexual arousal and climax, while men are more interested in watching naked bodies.

A new type of couple's pornography that appeals to both men and women is becoming increasingly available. These often combine story lines involving feelings and intimacy that are appealing to women along with graphic scenes that tend to be more appealing to men. Mutually stimulating pornography agreed to by both parties, either in the privacy of one's own bedroom watching DVDs or via an adult channel in a hotel rendezvous

Dr. Dorree Says:

You don't have to spend a lot of money or try a lot of strange things to spice up your sex life. Look around the house and use everyday things in a new ways to gently surprise each other. (Just stay away from the Noxzema!)

just for two (away from the kids and household chores) can be a luscious experience for both of you.

Sex Forever!

Whatever kind of sex you have, make it pleasurable, respectful, and fulfilling for both of you. And for the millionth time, allow us to remind you once again: Unless you are in a long-term, monogamous relationship, *please use those condoms!* Genital warts, herpes, HIV/AIDS, and all other sexually transmitted diseases have no age limit. You've made it this far. Now is the time to eat right, exercise, and protect yourself so you can enjoy the many pleasures of your body for as long as you possibly can.

Sex is a gift of life that we can enjoy for all of our years. As your body and life change, so does sex, but it doesn't have to disappear. Just when the media, Madison Avenue, and the medical world may be ready to count us out, we can blaze a new trail to our own authentic, evolving sexual selves in our 50s, 60s, 70s, 80s, and beyond. With years comes wisdom. We're not over the hill. We're out there on *top* of the hill, while the younger people behind us are still in the valley. And from the top of the hill we can now see more than they can imagine. We can see the truth: Sex never dies! Sex is the crossroads where the joys of the body meet the passions of the soul. Sex is the compass that leads us back to feel the vibrancy of life still coursing through our bodies, no matter what our bodies may become. Sex is our deepest selves remembering the primal force of life itself. Don't let declining hormones, relationship troubles, social expectations, or physical challenges permanently block you from that joy. Sex is your birthright, and as long as you are still here, it belongs to you.

Live as happily ever after as you can. Have as much fulfilling sex as you are able. We hope this book has helped you find your way. As pioneers you deserve to find the best sex yet.

TEN

YOUR OWN TRUTH, LIES, AND MUST-TRIES
Our Questions, Your Answers

Read through the following questions, divided by chapters, with three possible objectives in mind. First, these questions may help you better understand what sex means to you. Second, you can use these questions as a way to open up a conversation with your partner about how you both feel and what you each want. And finally, if you like, consider sharing your answers to these questions—or anything else you would like to ask or tell—with Dr. Dorree (anonymously and confidentially) by visiting her website at www.FiftyandFurthermore.com.

CHAPTER 1

YOU'RE STILL ROCKIN' AND WE DON'T MEAN IN A CHAIR!
Change Your Attitudes, Change Your Life

CHECK BOXES

Do you believe there is sex after 50? ❏ Yes ❏ No
Do you believe there is good sex after 50? ❏ Yes ❏ No

Do you believe everyone else has a better
sex life than you do?   ❏ Yes   ❏ No

Are you able to love, even if you don't
always like, everything about yourself?   ❏ Yes   ❏ No

Are you able to love, even if you don't
always like, everything about your partner?   ❏ Yes   ❏ No

Is sex a dull memory, and is that okay?   ❏ Yes   ❏ No

CHAPTER 2

SEX IS MORE THAN PROCREATION
As Hormones Wane, Sensuality Gains

Do you believe that as hormones wane,
sensuality can gain?   ❏ Yes   ❏ No

Do you believe that sex is only
worthwhile with intercourse?   ❏ Yes   ❏ No

Do you believe an orgasm is necessary
for good sex?   ❏ Yes   ❏ No

Do you believe people are born with
different levels of desire (libido)?   ❏ Yes   ❏ No

Do you believe that getting older
has any positive benefits?   ❏ Yes   ❏ No

CHAPTER 3

FEMALE MENOPAUSE AND SEX FOREVER
Keeping Your Juices Flowing

Do you believe women need
intimacy to have sex?   ❏ Yes   ❏ No

Do you believe a dry vagina is a necessary
part of getting older?   ❏ Yes   ❏ No

Is there a question you would love to ask
another woman about real-life sex after 50?   ❑ Yes   ❑ No

CHAPTER 4

MALE MEN-O-MORPH AND SEX FOREVER
Performance Power Customized

Do you believe that men need
intimacy to have sex?   ❑ Yes   ❑ No

Do you believe that a soft penis
can be your new joy-toy?   ❑ Yes   ❑ No

Is there a question you would love to
ask a man about real-life sex after 50?   ❑ Yes   ❑ No

CHAPTER 5

BETWEEN THE SHEETS
Great Sex from 50 to 100

Have you tried any new positions lately?   ❑ Yes   ❑ No
Do you believe if you don't use it, you will lose it?   ❑ Yes   ❑ No
Do you believe self-image makes a
difference in your sexual performance?   ❑ Yes   ❑ No
Do you believe your brain is the
most powerful sex organ?   ❑ Yes   ❑ No
Are you sure which is the bigger brain, the
one in the head or the one between the legs?   ❑ Yes   ❑ No
Do you believe that masturbation is okay?   ❑ Yes   ❑ No
Do you believe the media accurately
portrays you?   ❑ Yes   ❑ No

Do you believe the media accurately
portrays your values?   ❏ Yes ❏ No
Do you believe the media accurately
portrays your sex life?   ❏ Yes ❏ No
Do you believe that must-tries and how-to
techniques can change your bonus years?   ❏ Yes ❏ No
Is there anything you would change about
yourself in the bedroom?   ❏ Yes ❏ No

CHAPTER 6

OH, NO! WHERE DID MY LOVER GO?
Great Sex in a Long-term Relationship

Do you believe boring sex can be changed?   ❏ Yes ❏ No
Do you believe communication is
essential for good sex?   ❏ Yes ❏ No
Do you believe you can heat up
a cold relationship?   ❏ Yes ❏ No
Do you believe you can have
a good relationship without sex (intercourse)?   ❏ Yes ❏ No
Do you believe your partner should
read (know) your needs?   ❏ Yes ❏ No
Are you able to communicate your needs?   ❏ Yes ❏ No
Do you think you know what your
partner's emotional needs are?   ❏ Yes ❏ No
Do you think you know what your
partner's sexual needs are?   ❏ Yes ❏ No
Are you able to put yourself in your
partner's shoes?   ❏ Yes ❏ No

If you're in a long-term relationship
or marriage, is sex the same old same old,
and do you want it to change?   ❏ Yes ❏ No
Is there anything you would change
about your partner in the bedroom?   ❏ Yes ❏ No
Are you able to listen to your partner?   ❏ Yes ❏ No

CHAPTER 7

DATING AFTER FIFTY
Plenty of Fish in the Sea

Do you like giving gifts (from your heart,
that take time or that are tangible)?   ❏ Yes ❏ No
Do you like receiving gifts (from the heart,
gifts that take time, gifts that are tangible)? ❏ Yes ❏ No
Do you like physical touch?   ❏ Yes ❏ No
Do you like giving it?   ❏ Yes ❏ No
Do you like receiving it?   ❏ Yes ❏ No
Are you able to live and love alone?   ❏ Yes ❏ No
Can you have intercourse without a
meaningful relationship?   ❏ Yes ❏ No
Do you want a meaningful relationship
in order to have sex?   ❏ Yes ❏ No
Do you think love and marriage are best
together? Are you okay having one
without the other?   ❏ Yes ❏ No
Do you believe men and women
live on different planets?   ❏ Yes ❏ No
Do you believe same-sex relationships are okay? ❏ Yes ❏ No

CHAPTER 8

ILLNESSES, SCHMILLNESSES!
What to Do If You're No Longer an Acrobat

Do you believe you can have enjoyable
sex even with illness?   ❑ Yes   ❑ No

CHAPTER 9

THE GREAT JOY RIDE . . .
Something Fun for Everyone

Do you believe sex toys are okay?   ❑ Yes   ❑ No
Do you believe fantasizing during sex is okay?   ❑ Yes   ❑ No
Is there anything you would like to ask
or tell Dr. Dorree?   ❑ Yes   ❑ No

ASK DR. DORREE!

Have questions, comments, or stories
for Dr. Dorree Lynn?
Please submit them (anonymously, if you like) to
www.FiftyandFurthermore.com.
Look for her answers online or in her next book.

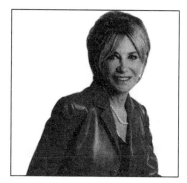

RESOURCES

Books

Berman, Laura, Ph.D. *Real Sex for Real Women*. New York: DK Publishing, 2008.

Block, Joel D. *Sex Over 50*. New York: Penguin Group, 1999.

Green, Gayle. *Insomniac*. Berkeley and Los Angeles: University of California Press, 2008.

Hendrix, Harville, Ph.D. *Getting the Love You Want*. New York: HarperPerennial, 1988.

Hendrix, Harville, Ph.D. *Keeping the Love You Find*. New York: Pocket Books, 1992.

Lynn, Dorree, Ph.D. *When the Man You Love Is Ill*. New York: Avalon Publishing Group, 2007.

McCarthy, Barry, and Emily McCarthy. *Rekindling Desire*. New York: Brunner-Routledge, 2003.

Northrup, Christiane, M.D. *The Wisdom of Menopause*. New York: Bantam Books, 2001.

Schnarch, David, Ph.D. *Passionate Marriage*. New York: Henry Holt and Company, 1997.

Sheehy, Gail. *Passages*. New York: E.P. Dutton and Co., Inc., 1974.

Trafford, Abigail. *As Time Goes By*. New York: Basic Books, Perseus Books Group, 2009.

Zilbergeld, Bernie, Ph.D. *The New Male Sexuality*. New York: Bantam Books, 1992.

Websites

www.AASECT.org. American Association of Sexuality, Educators, Counselors and Therapists.

www.AdamandEve.com.

www.Amazon.com. Sex Toys.

www.APA.org. American Psychological Association.

www.EvesGarden.com.

www.FiftyandFurthermore.com. Dr. Dorree Lynn's Questions, Answers, and Suggestions regarding sex and relationships, plus sex toys.

www.HotDogCollars.com. Pet supplies, like dog collars, can make inexpensive role-playing toys.

www.JimmyJane.com.

www.ThePenis.org. Info about the male genitals.

www.nwhn.org. National Women's Health Network. Information and resources on all aspects of women's health.

www.hpppa.org. Home Pleasure Party Plan Association, Inc. will arrange the equivalent of a Tupperware® party for sex toys.

REFERENCES

Altman, Alan M.D., and Suki Hanling, M.S.W., LICSW. *Sexuality in Midlife and Beyond*. Boston, MA: Harvard Health Publications, 2007.

American Association for Marriage and Family Therapy, http://www.aamft.org/.

American Psychological Association, www.apa.org.

Banner, Lois W. *In Full Flower*. New York: Alfred A. Knopf, 1992.

Bellman, Barbara, and Susan Goldstein. *Flirting After Fifty*. New York: Bloomington, iUniverse, Inc., 2008.

Berman, Laura, Ph.D. *Real Sex for Real Women*. New York: DK Publishing, 2008.

Berne, Eric, M.D. *Sex in Human Loving*. New York: Pocket Books, 1971.

Berne, Eric, M.D. *What Do You Say After You Say Hello?* New York: Bantam Books, 1972.

Block, Joel D. *Sex over 50*. New York: Penguin Group, 1999.

Bly, Robert. *Iron John*. Reading, MA: Addison-Wesley Publishing Company, Inc., 1990.

Butler, Robert N., M.D. and Myrna I. Lewis, Ph.D. *The New Love and Sex After 60*. New York: Ballantine Books, 1976.

Capra, Fritjof. *The Hidden Connections*. New York: Doubleday, 2002.

Center for Science in the Public Interest, http://www.cspinet.org/.

Centers for Disease Control and Prevention, www.CDC.gov.

Chapman, Gary. *The Five Love Languages*. Chicago: Northfield Publishing, 1992.

Childre, Doc, and Howard Martin, with Donna Beech. *The Heartmath Solution*. New York: Harper Collins Publishers, 1999.

Chua, Jasmin Malik. How to Tell True Blue Eco-Friendly Beauty

Products from No-Good Greenwashed Ones, May 4, 2009, http://planet green.discovery.com/fashion-beauty/elle-magazine-green-issue.html.

Colgrove, Melba, PhD., Harold H. Bloomfield, M.D., and Peter McWilliams. *How to Survive the Loss of a Love.* New York: Leo Press, 1967.

Cornell University Urology Department, http://www.cornellurology.com/.

Danielou, Alain. *The Complete Kama Sutra.* Rochester, VT: Park Street Press, 1994.

Deida, David. *Intimate Communion.* Deerfield Beach, Fl: Health Communications, Inc., 1995.

Doress-Worters, Paula B., and Diana Laskin Siegal. *The New Ourselves, Growing Older.* New York: Simon and Schuster, 1987.

Environmental Working Group's Cosmetic Safety Database, http://www.cosmeticsdatabase.com/index.php?

Estes, Clarissa Pinkola. *Women Who Run with Wolves.* New York, Ballantine Books, 1997.

Friday, Nancy. *Women on Top.* New York: Simon and Schuster, 1991.

Furman, Sue C. *Turning Point.* New York: Oxford University Press, 1995.

Generations 30, no. 3 (2006): 1–96.

Generations 32, no. 1 (2008): 1–88.

Germer, Fawn. *Hard Won Wisdom.* New York: The Berkley Publishing Group, 2001.

Green, Gayle. *Insomniac.* Berkeley and Los Angeles: University of California Press, 2008.

Greer, Germaine. *The Change.* New York: Fawcett Columbine, 1991.

Halonen, Jane S., and John W. Santrock. *Psychology: Contexts of Behavior.* Dubuque, IA: Times Mirror Higher Education Group, Inc., 1996.

Halpern, Howard M., Ph.D. *Finally Getting it Right.* New York: Bantam Books, 1994.

Harlow, B.L., L.A. Wise, M.W. Otto, C. Soares, and L.S. Cohen Lifetime history of depression and its influence on reproductive endocrine and menstrual cycle markers associated with perimenopause: The Harvard Study of Moods and Cycles. Arch *Gen Psych* 2003; 60:29–36

Harvard: *Walking: Your Steps to Health.* Harvard Men's Health Watch, August 2009.

Harvard: *What are Bioidentical Hormones?* Harvard Women's Health Watch, August 2006.

Hendrix, Harville, Ph.D. *Getting the Love You Want.* New York: HarperPerennial, 1988.

Hendrix, Harville, Ph.D. *Keeping the Love You Find.* New York: Pocket Books, 1992.

Hite, Shere. *The Hite Report.* New York: Macmillan Publishing Co., 1976.

Huey, Miranda. Skin Care Guide to Making Yours Eco-Friendly, http://www.greeniacs.com/GreeniacsGuides/Skin-Care-Guide-to-Making-Yours-Eco-Friendly.html.

Jon Paul, Chloe. *Entering the Age of Elegance.* Minneapolis, MI, Two Harbors Press, 2009.

Keen, Sam. *Fire in the Belly.* New York: Bantam Books, 1991.

Kinsey, Alfred Charles, Wardell B. Pomeroy, Clyde E. Martin, and Paul H. Gebhard. *Sexual Behavior in the Human Female.* Bloomington, IN: Indiana University Press, 1948.

Kinsey, Alfred Charles, Wardell Pomeroy, and Clyde E. Martin. *Sexual Behavior in the Human Male.* Bloomington, IN: Indiana University Press, 1948.

Kliger, Leah, MHA, and Deborah Nedelman, Ph.D. *Still Sexy After All These Years?* New York: Penguin Group, 2006.

Krupp, Charla. *How Not to Look Old.* New York: Springboard Press, 2008.

Levinson, Daniel J. *The Seasons of a Man's Life.* New York: Ballantine Books, 1978.

Leyner, Mark, and Billy Goldberg, M.D. *Why Do Men Have Nipples?* New York: Three Rivers Press, 2005.

Lindau, Stacy Tessler, M.D., MAPP, L. Philip Schumm, M.A., Edward O. Laumann, Ph.D., Wendy Levinson, M.D., Colm A. O'Muircheartaigh, Ph.D., and Linda J. Waite, Ph.D. "A Study of Sexuality and Health among Older Adults in the United States." *The New England Journal of Medicine,* Volume 357 (2007): 762–774.

Lynn, Dorree, Ph.D. *Getting Sane Without Going Crazy.* Xlibris Corporation, 2000.

Lynn, Dorree, Ph.D. "Is There a Therapist in the House?" *Voices: The Art and Science of Psychotherapy* 43, no. 1 (2007): 68–69.

Lynn, Dorree, Ph.D., and Isaacs Florence. *When the Man You Love is Ill.* New York: Avalon Publishing Group, 2007.

Malone, Thomas Patrick, M.D., and Patrick Thomas Malone, M.D. *The Art of Intimacy.* New York: Prentice Hall Press, 1987.

Manson, JoAnn E., M.D. *Hot Flashes, Hormones, and Your Health.* New York: McGraw Hill, 2007.

Mayo Clinic Special Report. *Mayo Clinic Health Solutions.* October 2007.

McCarthy, Barry, and Emily McCarthy. *Discovering Your Couple Sexual Style.* New York: Routledge, 2009.

McCarthy, Barry, and Emily McCarthy. *Rekindling Desire.* New York: Brunner-Routledge, 2003.

Mercola, Dr. Joseph. Secret Link Between Cigarettes and Cell Phones? September 2009. http://articles.mercola.com/sites/articles/archive/2009/09/29/More-Confirmation-That-Cell-Phones-Cause-Brain-Tumors.aspx.

Metz, Michael E. Ph.D., and Barry W. McCarthy. Ph.D. *Coping with Erectile Dysfunction.* Oakland, CA: New Harbinger Publications, Inc., 2004.

Montenegro, Xenia P. Ph.D., and Linda Fisher, Ph.D. "Sexuality at Midlife and Beyond." Washington, DC: AARP, 2005.

National Center for Health Statistics, http://www.cdc.gov/nchs/.

Northrup, Christiane, M.D. *The Wisdom of Menopause.* New York: Bantam Books, 2001.

Ogden, Gina, Ph.D. *The Heart and Soul of Sex.* Boston: Trumpeter, 2006.

Reuben, David M.D. *Everything You Always Wanted to Know About Sex.* New York: Van Rees Press, 1969.

Schachter-Shalomi, Zalman, and Ronald S. Miller. *From Age-ing to Sage-ing.* New York: Warner Books, 1995.

Schnarch, David, Ph.D. *Passionate Marriage.* New York: Henry Holt and Company, 1997.

Sheehy, Gail. *Passages.* New York: E.P. Dutton and Co., Inc., 1974.

Sheehy, Gail. *Sex and the Seasoned Woman.* New York: Ballantine Books, 2007.

Sheehy, Gail. *The Silent Passage.* New York: Random House, 1991.

Sheehy, Gail. *Understanding Men's Passages.* New York: Ballantine Books, 1998.

Sherfey, Mary Jane, M.D. *The Nature and Evolution of Female Sexuality.* New York: Vintage Books, 1966.

Sisley, Dr. Emily L., and Bertha Harris. *The Joy of Lesbian Sex.* New York: Crown Publishers, Inc., 1977.

Swallow, Wendy. *The Triumph of Love over Experience.* New York: Hyperion, 2004.

The Journal of the American Medical Association http://jama.ama-assn.org/.

Trafford, Abigail. *As Time Goes By*. New York: Basic Books, Perseus Books Group, 2009.

U.S. Surgeon General, http://www.surgeongeneral.gov/.

Vaughan, Peggy. *Musings on Life*. San Diego: Dialog Press, 2008.

Vaughan, Peggy. *The Monogamy Myth*. Newmarket Press, 2003.

Viorst, Judith. *Necessary Losses*. New York: Simon and Schuster, 1986.

Wald, Noreen. *Foxy Forever*. New York: St. Martin's Griffin, 2000.

Walsh, Mel. *Hot Granny*. San Francisco: Chronicle Books, 2007.

Weinstein, Sheila. *Moving to the Center of the Bed*. New York: Center of the Bed Publishing, 2009.

Westheimer, Dr. Ruth. *Sex for Dummies*. Hoboken, NJ: Wiley Publishing, Inc., 2007.

Wheat, Ed, M.D. *Love Life for Every Married Couple*. Grand Rapids, MI: Zondervan Publishing House, 1980.

Williams, Margery. *The Velveteen Rabbit*. Doubleday, 1958.

Winston, Sheri. *Women's Anatomy of Arousal*. Mango Garden Press. 2010.

Zgourides, George. *Human Sexuality*. New York: HarperCollins College Publishers, 1996.

Zilbergeld, Bernie, Ph.D. *Male Sexuality*. New York: Bantam Books, 1978.

INDEX

AARP Sexuality Study, 6,
201–202
accommodating sex, 123–124
Actis (penile band), 103
acupuncture
for facial care, 82
for menopausal symptoms, 61
for overall health, 262
for sleep disturbance, 252
for stress reduction, 165
addictions, 162, 175, 258, 286
adrenal hormones
adrenaline, 98
DHEA, 55, 59, 61
adrenaline, 98
adult sex shops, 274–276
adultery, 113–116, 230–232
affairs, 113–116, 230–232
age differences in relationships,
22, 228–230
aging, statistics, 5, 71
alcohol, 279, 280

Alka-Seltzer, 279
alternative treatments. *see also*
nutritional supplements
acupuncture, 61, 82, 165,
252, 262
massage, 47, 165, 252
meditation, 61, 118, 175, 252
for menopausal symptoms,
60–61
natural hormones, 60–61
use statistics, 262
yoga, 61, 118, 175, 252, 267
Alzheimer's disease, 249–250
anal desensitizers, 147
anal sex, 145–147
androgen, 58
anger/resentment, 123, 161,
176, 255
angry sex, 123, 176
antidepressants, 258–259, 266
anxiety/fear. *see also* sexual
performance anxiety

depression. *see also* moods *(cont'd from page 305)*
  perimenopause and, 257
  post heart attack, 240
  relationship challenges and, 161–162
  sexual problems and, 254–259
  studies, 47
DHEA, 55, 59, 61
diabetes, 243–244
dildos, 277
disease. *see* illness/disease
divorce, 111, 114, 258–259
doggie collars, 278
drugs. *see* medication
dryness, vaginal, 34, 52, 77–78, 224, 276

ejaculation
  controlling, 117
  intensity of, 127
  premature, 42, 90–92
  prostate enlargement and, 94–95
  surgical implants and, 104
  testosterone and, 88
electric tooth brush, 278
elevator dependency, 241
endorphins, 266
erectile dysfunction (ED)
  in advertising, 99–101
  causes, 102–103, 243–244, 254–256
  medical checkup, 105

medication cost, 100
medication side-effects, 100, 258–260
  as normal, 88
  treatment, 79, 85–86, 240–241, 244, 277
erections, 85–93. *see also* erectile dysfunction (ED); sexual performance anxiety
  adrenaline effect, 98
  anatomy of, 92–93
  depression/mood effect on, 254–259
  desire and, 100
  difficulties, 33, 105–107
  medications and, 98–99
Erexel (penile band), 103
Erikson, Erik, 21
erotic literature, 134, 270, 274, 286
erotic spots (physical), 76, 126
erotica, 124, 144, 192
Estes, Clarissa Pinkola, 79
estradiol, 54
estrogen. *see also* hormone replacement therapy (HRT)
  decline, 8, 35–36, 50–51, 57–58, 64–65
  estradiol, 54
  kinds of, 58
  localized boosters, 77
  in men, 87, 96
  phytoestrogens, 54
exercise
  for heart health, 239

women. *see also* menopause;
women's sexual anatomy
(cont'd from page 315)
masturbation, 36–37
new horizons, 79–80
relationship challenges, 62–66
role models, 69–71
same-sex relationships, 227–228
on sex after 50, 68–69
sex myths, 80
sexiness, 67–69
"wild" women, 80–81
Women Who Run with the Wolves
(Estes), 79
Women's Anatomy of Arousal
(Winston), 75–76

women's sexual anatomy. *see also*
clitoris; vagina
G-spot, 76
labia, 75
vulva, 38
Woodstock festival, 10–11

yeast infections, 244, 279
yoga
benefits of, 267
as sleep aide, 25
for stress reduction, 61, 118, 175
youth myth, 1–10, 14

zinc, 266